Forefoot Pain

Guest Editors

D. MARTIN CHANEY, DPM, MS
WALTER W. STRASH, DPM

CLINICS IN PODIATRIC MEDICINE AND SURGERY

www.podiatric.theclinics.com

Consulting Editor
THOMAS ZGONIS, DPM, FACFAS

October 2010 • Volume 27 • Number 4

SAUNDERS an imprint of ELSEVIER, Inc.

W.B. SAUNDERS COMPANY
A Division of Elsevier Inc.

1600 John F. Kennedy Boulevard ● Suite 1800 ● Philadelphia, Pennsylvania 19103-2899

http://www.theclinics.com

CLINICS IN PODIATRIC MEDICINE AND SURGERY Volume 27, Number 4
October 2010 ISSN 0891-8422, ISBN-13: 978-1-4377-2488-2

Editor: Patrick Manley
Developmental Editor: Donald Mumford

Clinics in Podiatric Medicine and Surgery (ISSN 0891-8422) is published quarterly by Elsevier Inc., 360 Park Avenue South, New York, NY 10010-1710. Months of issue are January, April, July, and October. Business and Editorial Offices: 1600 John F. Kennedy Blvd., Ste. 1800, Philadelphia, PA 19103-2899. Customer Service Office: 3251 Riverport Lane, Maryland Heights, MO 63043. Periodicals postage paid at New York, NY and additional mailing offices. Subscription prices are $270.00 per year for US individuals, $385.00 per year for US institutions, $137.00 per year for US students and residents, $324.00 per year for Canadian individuals, $477.00 for Canadian institutions, $384.00 for international individuals, $477.00 per year for international institutions and $193.00 per year for Canadian and foreign students/residents. To receive student/resident rate, orders must be accompanied by name of affiliated institution, date of term, and the *signature* of program/residency coordinator on institution letterhead. Orders will be billed at individual rate until proof of status is received. Foreign air speed delivery is included in all *Clinics* subscription prices. All prices are subject to change without notice. POSTMASTER: Send address changes to *Clinics in Podiatric Medicine and Surgery*, Elsevier Health Sciences Division, Subscription Customer Service, 3251 Riverport Lane, Maryland Heights, MO 63043. **Customer Service: 1-800-654-2452 (US). From outside of the US, call 314-447-8871. Fax: 314-447-8029. E-mail: JournalsCustomerService-usa@elsevier.com (for print support); JournalsOnlineSupport-usa@elsevier.com (for online support).**

Reprints. For copies of 100 or more of articles in this publication, please contact the Commercial Reprints Department, Elsevier Inc., 360 Park Avenue South, New York, NY 10010-1710. Tel.: 212-633-3812; Fax: 212-462-1935; E-mail: reprints@elsevier.com.

Clinics in Podiatric Medicine and Surgery is covered in *MEDLINE/PubMed (Index Medicus)* and *EMBASE/Excerpta Medica.*

Printed and bound by CPI Group (UK) Ltd, Croydon, CR0 4YY

Transferred to Digital Print 2011

CLINICS IN PODIATRIC MEDICINE AND SURGERY

Contributors

CONSULTING EDITOR

THOMAS ZGONIS, DPM, FACFAS
Director, Podiatric Surgical Residency and Reconstructive Fellowship Programs;
Chief, Division of Podiatric Medicine and Surgery; Associate Professor, Department
of Orthopedic Surgery, The University of Texas Health Science Center at San Antonio,
San Antonio, Texas

GUEST EDITORS

D. MARTIN CHANEY, DPM, MS
Private Practice - Alamo Family Foot & Ankle Care, San Antonio, Texas

WALTER W. STRASH, DPM
Private Practice - Alamo Family Foot & Ankle Care, San Antonio, Texas

AUTHORS

WILLIAM R. ADAMS II, DPM, FACFAS
Diplomate, American Board of Podiatric Surgery; Director, Wound Care Center,
Jackson Purchase Medical Center; Private Practice, Advanced Foot and Ankle Clinic,
Mayfield, Kentucky

ERIC A. BARP, DPM, FACFAS
Private Practice, Des Moines, Iowa

IOANNIS S. BENETOS, MD
Third Department of Orthopaedics, Athens University Medical School, Athens, Greece

CHRISTOPHER BIBBO, DO, DPM, FACS, FACFAS, FAAOS, FACLES, FACLES
Chief Foot & Ankle Service, Department of Orthopaedics, Marshfield Clinic, Marshfield,
Wisconsin; Clinical Instructor, St Joseph Hospital/North Chicago VAMC PM&S-36
Podiatry Residency, Chicago, Illinois

DONALD E. BUDDECKE, DPM, FACFAS
Private Practice, Omaha, Nebraska

CATHERINE A. CASTEEL, DPM
Department of Podiatry, Hunt Regional Medical Center of Greenville, Greenvillle, Texas

D. MARTIN CHANEY, DPM, MS
Private Practice, Alamo Family Foot & Ankle Care, San Antonio, Texas

FRANCIS DERK, DPM
Chief, Podiatry Division, Department of Surgery, Audie L. Murphy Veterans Affairs
Hospital, San Antonio, Texas

BRIAN E. DE YOE, DPM
Department of Orthopedics, Metroplex Foot and Ankle, Dallas, Texas

ROZALIA DIMITRIOU, MD
First Department of Orthopaedics, Athens University Medical School, Athens, Greece

KYLE FIALA, DPM
Resident PGY-2, Podiatric Medicine and Surgical Residency, Truman Medical Center, Lakewood, Kansas City, Missouri

ADAM GOLDKIND, DPM
PGY-3 Chief Resident, St Joseph Hospital/North Chicago VAMC PM&S-36 Podiatry Residency; Department of Podiatry, St Joseph Hospital, Chicago, Illinois

JAMES GOOD, DPM, FACFAS
Residency Director, Podiatric Medicine and Surgical Residency, Truman Medical Center, Lakewood, Kansas City, Missouri

LCDR MONIQUE C. GOURDINE-SHAW, DPM
United States Naval Academy, Annapolis, Maryland; Veteran Affairs Maryland Healthcare Systems, Baltimore, Maryland

LELAND JAFFE, DPM
PGY-3 Chief Resident, St Joseph Hospital/North Chicago VAMC PM&S-36 Podiatry Residency; Department of Podiatry, St Joseph Hospital, Chicago, Illinois

SEAN KERSH, DPM
Podiatric Surgical Resident, Division of Podiatric Medicine and Surgery, Department of Orthopaedic Surgery, The University of Texas Health Science Center at San Antonio, San Antonio, Texas

DEMETRIOS S. KORRES, MD
Third Department of Orthopaedics, Athens University Medical School, Athens, Greece

SHIRMEEN LAKHANI, DPM
Podiatric Surgical Resident, Division of Podiatric Medicine and Surgery, Department of Orthopaedic Surgery, The University of Texas Health Science Center at San Antonio, San Antonio, Texas

BRADLEY M. LAMM, DPM
Head of Foot and Ankle Surgery, Director of the Foot and Ankle Deformity Correction Fellowship, International Center for Limb Lengthening, Rubin Institute for Advanced Orthopedics, Sinai Hospital of Baltimore, Baltimore, Maryland

ANDREAS F. MAVROGENIS, MD
First Department of Orthopaedics, Athens University Medical School, Athens, Greece

PANAYIOTIS J. PAPAGELOPOULOS, MD, DSc
First Department of Orthopaedics, Athens University Medical School, Athens, Greece

MATTHEW A. POLK, DPM
Resident, Saint Joseph Hospital, Chicago, Illinois

ROGER RACZ, DPM
Great Falls Clinic, Great Falls, Montana

CRYSTAL L. RAMANUJAM, DPM
Fellow, Postgraduate Research and Clinical Instructor, Division of Podiatric Medicine and Surgery, Department of Orthopaedic Surgery, The University of Texas Health Science Center at San Antonio, San Antonio, Texas

ALEX SIKORSKI, MD
Department of Podiatry, Malteser Foot Center, Reinbach, Germany

WALTER W. STRASH, DPM
Private Practice, Alamo Family Foot & Ankle Care, San Antonio, Texas

THOMAS ZGONIS, DPM, FACFAS
Director, Podiatric Surgical Residency and Reconstructive Fellowship Programs; Chief, Division of Podiatric Medicine and Surgery; Associate Professor, Department of Orthopedic Surgery, The University of Texas Health Science Center at San Antonio, San Antonio, Texas

Contents

Complications associated with digital and lesser metatarsal surgical procedures have been well documented in the literature. These complications may stem from systemic medical, structural, biologic, biomechanical, or iatrogenic causes. The surgeon must be cognizant of all potential complications, including ways to prevent them from occurring and how to manage them when they do occur. This article discusses preventative measures through the preoperative evaluation of the patient, and examines the subsets of complications that may occur after lesser ray surgery that pose a particular management challenge, as well as special complications specific to particular operative techniques.

The purpose of this article is to address the isolated causes of osseous central metatarsalgia that are related to an elongated metatarsal and brachymetatarsalgia. The authors focus on surgically addressing shortened and elongated metatarsals, surgical complications, and revisional surgery.

Puncture wounds are common injuries of the foot. Although most puncture wounds are benign, devastating complications are possible without adequate treatment. These injuries can occur in all age groups and in various circumstances. Early diagnosis and appropriate medical and surgical management is paramount in achieving successful outcomes.

Morton neuroma is a common source of forefoot pain. This condition is more correctly termed as interdigital nerve compression and is not a true neuroma. Although Morton neuroma is a common diagnosis, debate exists as to the best surgical and nonsurgical treatments. This article discusses the pathogenesis, diagnosis, nonsurgical and surgical management, and surgical complications of this common disorder.

these fractures can cause a significant inconvenience to the patient. With the exception of fifth metatarsal base fractures, little standardization is available for the treatment of metatarsal fractures. Controversy still exists regarding the proper treatment of various patient populations for junctional fifth metatarsal fractures. This article discusses the fractures of the first, central, and fifth metatarsals, as well as the treatment for the same.

Fifth toe positional problems typically cause irritation with various forms of footgear. The position of the toe causes irritation against the toe box of the shoe. This article discusses the physical examination of various fifth toe deformities along with the different approaches of arthroplasty that are used to correct the deformity and the management of complications that arise from the correction procedures.

Current Concepts and Techniques in Foot and Ankle Surgery

Juxta-articular osteoid osteomas of the ankle are rare and tend to have an atypical presentation. Because of the proximity to the joint, patients experience symptoms that may delay or mislead the diagnosis. This article presents a 33-year-old man with juxta-articular osteoid osteoma of the talar neck. The correct diagnosis was delayed for 2 years; the patient was initially misdiagnosed and treated for ankle sprain and anterior ankle impingement. Surgical excision of the lesion was performed with excellent results. Juxta-articular osteoid osteomas should be considered in the differential diagnosis of persistent ankle pain in teenagers and young adults who do not respond to treatment directed at more common conditions.

Squamous cell carcinoma of the foot is a common malignant neoplasm with a high potential for metastasis. Squamous cell carcinoma arising in chronic osteomyelitis has been widely reported; however, its presence in combination with acute osteomyelitis of the foot is not well known. This article presents such a case that demonstrates the importance of early recognition with appropriate management for limb salvage and successful oncologic outcome.

FORTHCOMING ISSUES

RECENT ISSUES

THE CLINICS ARE NOW AVAILABLE ONLINE!

Access your subscription at:
www.theclinics.com

Foreword

Forefoot Pain

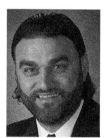

Thomas Zgonis, DPM, FACFAS
Consulting Editor

Forefoot pain is one of the most common problems encountered in our foot and ankle practices. Many disorders affect the forefoot region, often making diagnosis and treatment a challenge. For example, hallux abducto valgus is very common and often treated with surgery. The unique aspect of the surgical treatment of hallux abducto valgus is the fact that so many different procedures and techniques are utilized to successfully address this common deformity. In addition, in order to address this surgical entity, a thorough understanding of forefoot biomechanics and how it relates to rearfoot/ankle and the lower extremity is paramount in diagnosing and treating most common forefoot deformities.

In this issue, Drs Chaney and Strash have invited a great panel to share their expertise in forefoot surgery. Articles focus on understanding lesser metatarsal osteotomies, digital surgery, peripheral nerve entrapment, brachymetatarsia, and puncture wounds. The complex nature of various forefoot deformities is addressed in detail along with the etiologic factors and treatment of neurogenic forefoot pathologies. These conditions may require additional diagnostic and medical imaging along with a thorough understanding of the forefoot biomechanics and neurogenic pain.

This issue also marks my second year as a Consulting Editor for the *Clinics in Podiatric Medicine and Surgery*. I am honored and committed to continue bringing innovative topics to be covered in the *Clinics in Podiatric Medicine and Surgery*. Finally, I want to thank all the contributors and prestigious editorial board members for their continuous efforts and contributions.

Thomas Zgonis, DPM, FACFAS
Division of Podiatric Medicine and Surgery
Department of Orthopaedic Surgery
The University of Texas Health Science Center at San Antonio
7703 Floyd Curl Drive – MSC 7776
San Antonio, TX 78229, USA

E-mail address:
zgonis@uthscsa.edu

Clin Podiatr Med Surg 27 (2010) xiii
doi:10.1016/j.cpm.2010.08.003
0891-8422/10/$ – see front matter © 2010 Elsevier Inc. All rights reserved.

podiatric.theclinics.com

Preface

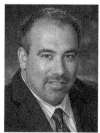 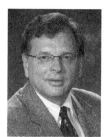

D. Martin Chaney, DPM, MS   Walter W. Strash, DPM
Guest Editors

I would like to thank all of the authors for their hard work on this issue. I think each article will provide new insight to problems seen frequently in our practices to improve our patients' outcomes. Physicians reading this issue have all worked hard to obtain the privilege to treat another human being's pain and ailments. Our patients' outcomes are our number one priority. Our actions can have profound effects on our patients' quality of life.

Life is short. As physicians, our patients, our family, and our selves deserve the attention to detail to make this short life as enjoyable and productive as possible. Leave no regrets knowing you did all you could or ever wanted to.

D. Martin Chaney, DPM, MS

Walter W. Strash, DPM
Private Practice - Alamo Family Foot & Ankle Care
San Antonio, TX, USA

E-mail addresses:
marty.chaney@gmail.com (D.M. Chaney)
podcanuck@aol.com (W.W. Strash)

Clin Podiatr Med Surg 27 (2010) xv
doi:10.1016/j.cpm.2010.08.002   **podiatric.theclinics.com**
0891-8422/10/$ — see front matter © 2010 Elsevier Inc. All rights reserved.

Complications of Digital and Lesser Metatarsal Surgery

Christopher Bibbo, DO, DPM[a,b,]*, Leland Jaffe, DPM[b,c],
Adam Goldkind, DPM[b,c]

KEYWORDS

- Complications • Digital • Metatarsal • Surgery
- Infection • Nonunion

Deformity of the digits and lesser metatarsals is a common surgical problem presenting to the foot and ankle surgeon. Although elective operative management is usually straightforward, even the most routine cases carry the risk of surgical complication, spanning from the simple to the devastating. Numerous complications associated with many of the common forefoot procedures have been well documented in the literature, as well as from observations by individual surgeons in the course of thousands of operative procedures. Although frequently defined as iatrogenic, complications may more often be related to systemic medical, structural, biologic, or biomechanical causes. Although sound clinical judgment and surgical skills can help prevent many intraoperative complications, a thorough preoperative evaluation of the patient is critical for a successful surgical outcome. This article discusses preventative measures through the preoperative evaluation of the patient, and examines the subsets of complications that may occur after lesser ray surgery that pose a particular management challenge, as well as special complications specific to particular operative techniques.

RISK FACTORS AND MEDICAL COMORBIDITIES

Proper patient selection is essential for elective forefoot reconstructive surgery. Successful surgical outcomes not only depend on the surgeon's technique in the operating suite, but assessing the patient's background for proper medical decision

[a] Foot and Ankle Service, Department of Orthopaedics, Marshfield Clinic, 1000 North Oak Avenue, Marshfield, WI 54449, USA
[b] St Joseph Hospital/North Chicago VAMC PM&S-36 Podiatry Residency, Chicago, IL, USA
[c] Department of Podiatry, St Joseph Hospital, 2900 North Lake Shore Drive, Chicago, IL 60657, USA
* Corresponding author. Department of Orthopaedics, Marshfield Clinic, 1000 North Oak Avenue, Marshfield, WI 54449.
E-mail address: bibbo.christopher@marshfieldclinic.org

Clin Podiatr Med Surg 27 (2010) 485–507
doi:10.1016/j.cpm.2010.06.001
0891-8422/10/$ – see front matter © 2010 Published by Elsevier Inc.

podiatric.theclinics.com

making also increases the probability of achieving better healing in the postoperative setting. It is therefore in the best interest of the physician to gather a detailed history and physical before decision making and use the data collected from the interview to assess the possible complications that could hinder optimal outcomes. When considering the entire patient picture, modifiable and nonmodifiable risk factors play a role in proper healing and the success of the treatment (**Box 1**).

The Effect of Diabetes on Complications

Diabetes is a nonmodifiable risk factor that presents unique challenges to the podiatric surgeon. Diabetes has frequently been linked to complications associated with bone and soft-tissue healing.[1] Before elective forefoot surgery, patients with diabetes need to be informed of their increased risk factors including, but not limited to, infection, delayed union, nonunion, and impaired wound healing. Strict glycemic control has been shown to limit the incidence of these negative surgical outcomes in patients with diabetes. Hyperglycemia as a result of diabetes results in enzymatic glycoslyation of structural proteins, producing advanced glycoslyation end products (AGEs). These AGEs can attach to inflammatory reactants, basement membranes, and collagen, and negatively affect wound and bone healing by impairing the body's natural healing cascade.[1] AGEs also increase low-density lipoprotein (LDL) levels, accelerating the development of atherosclerosis, affecting large- and medium-sized vessels.[2] In addition, specific tissues such as blood vessels, kidneys, and eyes do not require insulin for glucose transport. In these specific tissues, hyperglycemia shifts the polyol pathway to the production of sorbital, resulting in decreased myoinositol levels and cell damage.[1] These consequences from the hyperglycemic state result in angiopathy, immunopathy, and neuropathy, all of which can delay the healing process. It is the responsibility of the surgeon to ensure that the patient is in a euglycemic state and that the hemoglobin A1C (HgA1C) level is within normal limits before proceeding with elective operations of the forefoot.

Immunopathy as a complication of uncontrolled diabetes results in increased rates of bacterial colonization and local infection. Bacteria release metalloproteinases, which break down fibrin and growth factors necessary for wound healing.[1] Furthermore, angiopathy can leave the patient with diabetes in a hypoxic state, increasing

---

Box 1
Modifiable and nonmodifiable risk factors

Modifiable risk factors

Tobacco

Alcohol

Nutritional deficiencies

(Patient compliance)

Nonmodifiable risk factors

Diabetes mellitus

Rheumatoid arthritis

Collagen vascular disease

Osteoporosis

the potential for wound healing complications. Hypoxia can limit fibroblast proliferation as well as the deposition of collagen, further limiting wound healing.[1] In a clinical study evaluating 31 patients with lower extremity fractures, Loder[3] found that the time to fracture union in diabetics was 163% that of patients who do not have diabetes. These factors must be considered when considering elective operations on patients with diabetes.

Rheumatoid Arthritis and Complications

Patients with rheumatoid arthritis (RA) present a challenge to the foot and ankle surgeon, often presenting with disabling foot deformities that may require reconstructive forefoot surgery. By the nature of their disease process, people with RA are often considered compromised patients with an increased risk for postoperative infections and delayed bone and soft-tissue healing. These patients often require numerous surgical procedures to correct their foot deformities, further increasing the risk of postoperative complications. Although the disease process begins initially with immune complexes in the synovial membrane causing an inflammatory synovitis, progression of RA results in the hyperplastic synovium, or pannus, to cause cartilage and osseous erosions. Periarticular osteoporosis is a commonly documented result of RA, but it is inconclusive if RA results in a generalized condition of osteoporosis. There seems to be a correlation between increased radiological RA destruction and low bone mineral density at the hip as determined by dual energy x-ray absorptiometry (DEXA) scan analysis.[4] This study implies a relationship between the severity/progression of RA, the medications to treat the disease, and the development of decreased bone mineral density. Thus, careful radiographic scrutiny of the quality of bone mineralization must be performed, and appropriate steps taken to ensure that instrumentation and bone healing augmentation are implemented. The podiatric surgeon should be aware of the detrimental effects of RA on bone and soft-tissue healing before proceeding with elective reconstructive surgery. Bibbo and colleagues[5] documented a 32% complication rate of 104 patients undergoing 725 procedures for rheumatoid reconstructive foot and ankle surgery. Whether RA medications should be discontinued before elective surgery remains debated. Those who have identifiable risks or a proven history of wound healing problems should be considered to have their RA medications held in the immediate perioperative period.[6]

Wound Healing and Infectious Complications

Wound healing complications from foot surgery can present difficult complications for the patient and surgeon. Difficulties healing surgical incisions can stem from systemic, mechanical, iatrogenic, or patient noncompliance. Problems from wound healing can range from mild dehiscence to frank necrosis along the incision site. Wound healing can be divided into 3 phases. The inflammatory phase occurs during the first 6 days, during which time the fibrin clot forms in the wound site. Neutrophils, monocytes, and platelets are active during this phase. The next phase is the fibroblastic proliferation and angiogenesis phase that occurs from day 6 to day 14 to day 21. It is during this time that epithelial cell growth and collagen production occurs. The development of myofibroblasts marks the beginning of the last phase, or remodeling phase, during which time the tensile strength of the wound is increased.[7] Disruption during any of these phases can negatively affect the healing process, such as in uncontrolled patients with diabetes who are unable to naturally progress through the first 2 stages.[8]

Surgeon technique and preoperative considerations are also critical to minimizing the risk of soft-tissue complications and infections. In a study performed by Bibbo and colleagues,[9] different preoperative skin preparations were compared including chlorhexidine scrub and isopropyl alcohol paint versus povidone-iodine scrub and paint. Data from this study revealed that the chlorhexidine and alcohol scrub had a prolonged bactericidal action and a greater reduction in the number of common bacterial flora (including staphylococcus and diptheroid species) found on the foot compared with the povidone-iodine scrub and paint. Also preoperatively, the foot should be examined for ulcerative lesions or any other breaks in the skin. Bacterial colonization in ulcerative lesions can potentially lead to postoperative infection. In general, prophylactic preoperative antibiotics are still the standard of care for all clean, elective surgical forefoot cases.

Postoperative patient observation and follow-up are keys in detecting early signs of complications. In the senior author's practice, all patients are seen at a minimum of 7 days after operation. Patients admitted overnight routinely have dressing changes before discharge when even the slightest discomfort is present associated with a dressing or postoperative therapeutic intervention. Even routine practices in postoperative patient care may be the source of complications. An example of this is documented in a case review of 2 patients developing frostbite of the feet from routine postoperative cryotherapy. The first patient was discharged home with an ankle cryo/cuff status after bilateral bunion surgery, and the second patient received a continuous ice-flow device status after elective first ray and digitial surgery. These patients were exposed to prolonged uninterrupted cryotherapy for 4 to 7 days, resulting in extensive soft-tissue necrosis, compartment syndromes, and limb-threatening frostbite injuries.[10] This example highlights how routine postoperative protocols can lead to severe complications.

The presence of a postoperative hematoma or infection can also negatively affect the healing process. Potential for hematoma formation is increased with the creation of a surgical void or failure of proper hemostasis, and the use of an open or closed drain can help minimize this risk. Patients who are medically anticoagulated pose a particular risk for troublesome postoperative hematoma formation. Hematomas mechanically disrupt the integrity of the incision site and serve as nidus for infection.[11] Once bacterial load along an incision site transitions from contamination to colonization to frank infection, numerous conditions exist that impair wound healing. Bacterial infection negatively affects the healing cascade by activating an alternate complement pathway and significantly extending the inflammatory phase or first phase of wound healing. Bacteria release enzymes and metalloproteinases that have been shown to degrade collagen and fibrin and inhibit essential growth factors.[1] Bacteria also compete for oxygen and nutrients in the wound, resulting in a hypoxic state. Hypoxic conditions produce lactic acid causing further release of proteolytic enzymes destructive to wound healing.[11] These complications can be minimized by meticulous surgical technique, proper hemostasis, and maintaining proper aseptic technique. It is the investigators' recommendation to use drains liberally when large dead spaces are created or if a patient is to receive anticoagulation in the perioperative period. Drains are maintained after operations until less than 10 mL of drainage is noted during 2 consecutive 8-hour shifts. Once a hematoma is recognized, it may require compression dressings, sterile aspiration, or surgical evacuation (**Fig. 1**).

Wound dehiscence and postoperative infections, once identified, should be aggressively managed in a timely fashion. Radiographic evaluation may reveal peri-implant lucency, as well as changes in soft-tissue density consistent with gas or abscess formation. A white blood cell count, erythrocyte sedimentation rate, as well as C-reactive protein (CRP) should be obtained for comparing future trends with baseline values. CRP has been suggested to be more specific for infected implants and

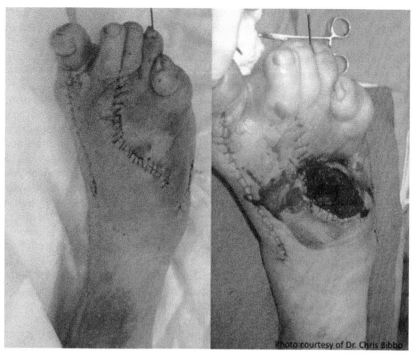

Fig. 1. Postoperative hematoma after elective metatarsal osteotomies for skew-foot deformity in an anticoagulated patient. This condition required surgical evacuation and negative pressure therapy.

hardware.[12] The surgeon must correlate laboratory and radiographic changes with clinical findings to formulate a proper treatment plan for the patient. Definitive antibiotic coverage should be based on direct specimen cultures and sensitivities.

Smoking has a detrimental effect on the respiratory and cardiovascular systems, but smoking also can negatively affect the musculoskeletal system. Cigarette smoke contains numerous toxins that can significantly affect tissue metabolism. Nicotine contained in cigarette smoke releases catecholamines, resulting in vasoconstriction and decreased perfusion to bone and soft tissue. Nicotine also can adversely affect circulation by decreasing levels of prostacyclin, a potent vasodilator.[13] A compromise in circulation decreases the delivery of critical growth factors that are required for adequate bone and soft-tissue healing. Cigarette smoke also contains carbon monoxide, which binds to hemoglobin with a higher affinity than oxygen, further decreasing the amount of oxygen delivered at the tissue level.[13] A study performed by Krannitz and colleagues[14] compared the rate of bone healing in elective forefoot surgery in smokers, nonsmokers, and second-hand smokers. The average rate of bone healing after an Austin osteotomy in smokers was 120 days, versus 69 days and 78 days for nonsmokers and second-hand smokers respectively. Although smoking clearly negatively affects bone healing, the time frame in which cessation of smoking improves the rates of bone union is uncertain. It is the investigators' standard protocol to encourage patients to discontinue smoking before elective forefoot surgery.

Alcohol abuse has also been proved to delay bone healing. Alcohol is cytotoxic to human mesenchymal stem cells that are determined for osteogenesis.[15] In the cascade of bone healing, bone morphogenic proteins (BMPs) bind to mesenchymal stem cells, causing the stem cells to differentiate into osteoblasts, and ultimately results in bone healing. A disruption in this cascade from chronic alcohol abuse can be detrimental to the bone healing process by impeding stem cell differentiation.[15]

In addition to alcohol abuse and smoking, many other situations exist that categorize patients as high-risk surgical candidates for osseous healing. These situations include, but are not limited to, revision surgery, chronic infections, suboptimal vascular supply, and history of delayed or nonunions.[16] Osseous insult, whether surgical or traumatic, causes the body to proceed through the natural healing cascade. Stages of osseous healing proceed from inflammation, to regeneration, and finally tissue remodeling; disruption along the healing cascade can lead to a delayed or nonunion. During the postoperative period, the surgeon should be performing routine radiographic examinations of the surgical site to assess the progress of bone healing. In general, the time line for declaring a delayed osseous union is 8 weeks, although variations occur among anatomic regions within the foot. When a delayed union is declared, the surgeon should strongly consider using a bone stimulator and immobilization with limited weight bearing on the involved extremity. At 12 weeks after operation, if radiographic progression of bone healing has ceased, the diagnosis of osseous nonunion can be made. At this point in the postoperative period the surgeon should reassess the preoperative risk factors, rule out an infectious process, and consider revision of fixation technique along with bone grafting or orthobiologic augmentation of the nonunion site. Autogenous bone grafts contain osteoconductive, osteoinductive, and osteogenic properties, making this the gold standard for bone healing augmentation. Emerging advancements in orthobiologics have introduced other options to augment bone healing, such as Infuse bone graft (recombinant BMP type 2 [rhBMP-2]), platelet rich plasma (PRP), and bone marrow aspirate.[17–19] BMPs are naturally occurring inducible proteins belonging to the transforming growth factor-β (TGF-β) supergene family. BMPs are highly osteoinductive materials that help bone advance through the natural healing cascade.[20] PRPs act as a reservoir for critical growth factors required for proper bone healing, and have been shown to decrease the time to osseous union. Bone marrow aspirate contains osteoconductive and osteoinductive properties, augmenting the healing cascade.[21] However, using orthobiologic technology does not supplement proper surgical technique and stable fixation. Revising a diagnosed osseous nonunion may require prolonged immobilization and revising fixation techniques, combined with using orthobiologic technology.

Implant Failure and Management

Appropriate preoperative considerations must be made regarding implantable hardware for those procedures requiring internal fixation in patients with suboptimal bone density or obesity. Traditional plates create compression at the plate-bone interface and rely on this friction for stability. With axial loading, the screws can begin to piston, decreasing this plate-bone friction and causing plate loosening.[22] Appropriate implant selection takes into consideration the procedure being performed, patient age, bone stock, bone size, and postoperative weight-bearing protocols. Although locking plate technology may provide enhanced rigidity of bone-implant constructs, if improperly used, especially in patients with poor bone density, failure may still be catastrophic. These plates do not allow unrestricted weight bearing for the patient in the postoperative period, and are still subject to failure if implant tolerances are exceeded (**Fig. 2**). It is imperative to formulate a safe and realistic postoperative plan for these patients in order to minimize the risk of hardware failure and associated

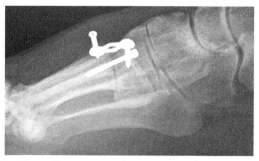

Fig. 2. Failed locking plate after metatarsal osteotomy. Flaws within locking plate technology are still emerging.

malunion, delayed union, or nonunion. Despite the documented benefits of locking plate technology, locking plates are not a substitute for good surgical technique.

Implants used for lesser metatarsal and digital surgery can be a source of complications for the foot and ankle surgeon. Implants can mechanically fail, cause a metal sensitivity reaction, or act as a surface for biofilm formation resulting in acute or latent infection. Metal sensitivity is a well-documented phenomenon that can create a potential for implant failure. Once a metallic orthopedic device is implanted, the body's natural biologic enzymes cause corrosion of the implant, releasing ions. These ions form complexes with proteins within the body that can activate the immune system causing a hypersensitivity reaction.[23] The prevalence of nickel sensitivity is highest among the general population at 14%, with other metal alloys causing a sensitivity reaction in about 10% to 15% of the population.[23] Hypersensitivity reactions to implants can be either a type-I cell-mediated immediate response (minutes), or, more commonly, a type-IV delayed-type hypersensitivity (DTH) reaction. Patch testing is traditionally used to test for DTH reactions, but there is doubt as to the relevance of a positive patch test in predicting the body's immune response to metallic implants.[23] In the senior author's experience, metal sensitivity is a rare phenomenon but, when it occurs, it can mimic an intense inflammatory reaction or infection. Diagnosis is generally on clinical grounds, rendered after a thorough, systematic process of elimination of other causes (eg, infection).Implant removal may ultimately be required.

Implants may also act as a nidus for infection. Implants have the potential to negatively affect the body's local immune response, ostensibly through the release of metal ions (ex-titanium). Additionally, particular metals/metal compounds possess nanostructures that may inhibit or encourage bacterial colonization of the implant and form a polyglycolic slime layer (glycocalyx), effectively inhibiting antibiotic penetration.[24] It has recently been recognized that implant infections are often caused by methicillin-resistant coagulase-negative staphylococcus (*Staphylococcus epidermidis*), once considered a mere contamination of cultures rather than the true infection it is now recognized to cause. Thus, it has been recommended that, in the management of patients with known or suspected implant infections, or those patients at risk for developing implant infections, surgical prophylaxis should entertain the use of vancomycin 1 hour before skin incision.[24]

Identifying infected hardware and deciding on the appropriate management can be challenging for the surgeon. Implant infection or failure can stem from numerous causes including poor surgical technique, inherent risks or specific surgical procedures, or hematogenous spread of bacteria. A thorough preoperative history can identify potential risk factors such as a recent upper respiratory tract infection, urinary tract infection, or dental procedure, all of which could hematogenously infect implanted hardware. In addition, certain surgical techniques have an inherent risk for infection. For example, using a percutaneous Kirschner wire for fixation of digital arthrodesis increases the risk for postoperative pin-tract infection versus using a buried Kirschner wire as internal fixation.[25] Kirschner wire fixation can also potentially lead to additional complications, such as metatarsal head avascular necrosis if placed across the metatarsalphalangeal joint (MPJ), especially with repeated attempts at appropriate alignment (**Fig. 3**). Failed fusion attempts of the lesser MPJs are difficult and may require bone grafting. In properly selected cases, salvage may also be suited to metatarsal head resection or unipolar joint resurfacing (**Fig. 4**).

Management of hardware infection has been a subject of debate in recent literature. Initial antibiotic therapy should target *Staphylococcus aureus* and *S epidermidis*, the 2 most common bacteria resulting in postoperative infections.[12,26] Initial use of broad-spectrum antibiotic therapy could potentially lead to multidrug resistant bacterial infections. Treatment of infected implants also may require surgical incision and drainage and possible hardware removal. The decision to remove implanted hardware should be based on several factors. First, the surgeon should determine whether the underlying fracture or osteotomy is biomechanically stable and has healed.[27] If the bone is well healed, it is the investigators' recommendation to remove the internal hardware and initiate antibiotic therapy. The decision-making process becomes difficult with an unstable osseous segment with overlying skin and soft-tissue infection. However, grossly infected implants with deep abscess formation and purulent

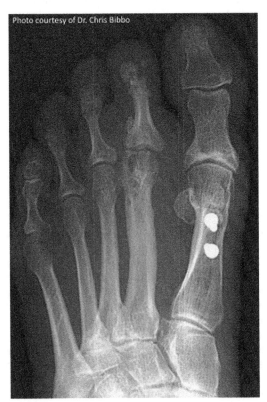

Photo courtesy of Dr. Chris Bibbo

Fig. 3. Second ray osteomyelitis and avascular necrosis secondary to Kirschner wire fixation.

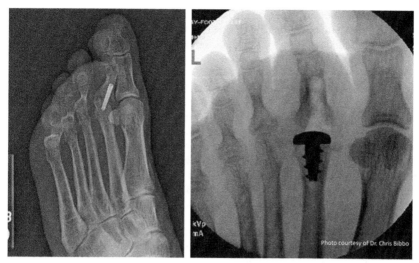

Fig. 4. Failed attempted second metatarsophalangeal fusion referred for pain and deformity (*left panel*). Salvage with second metatarsophalangeal joint hemiarthroplasty, with resolution of pain and improved motion (*right panel*).

drainage often require removal of the implant. Because of the glycocalyx layer on the retained infected hardware, the implant remains a nidus for infection and should be removed.[24,28] If the underlying bone remains unstable after removal of the implanted hardware, the surgeon should strongly consider stabilizing the osseous segments with an external fixator.

Lesser MPJ silastic implants can also present specific complications. Silastic implants have been documented to cause detritic synovitis because of degeneration of the implant. A reactive synovitis can develop intraarticularly secondary to microscopic particulate shards from the silicone implant.[29] Silastic implants serve as joint spacers and have an increased potential to fail when placed into a load-bearing joint such as the second MPJ. Failure of these implants not only can result in an inflammatory synovitis but can also destabilize the joint. Potential salvage procedures of a failed silastic implant include hemiarthroplasty of the metatarsal head or arthrodesis of the involved MPJ (see **Fig. 4**).

Acute Digital Correction of Long-standing Toe Deformities

The elderly, and especially patients with RA commonly present to the podiatrist's office with disabling forefoot pathologies and often elect for forefoot surgical reconstructive surgery. Digital deformities are a common manifestation of the disease requiring podiatric assessment. In a study by Michelson and colleagues,[30] 94% of patients with RA had painful symptoms related to the foot and ankle some time after their RA diagnosis, and 28% of these patients had specific forefoot problems. Disruption of the collateral ligaments and capsule of the lesser MPJs secondary to inflammatory synovitis can lead to instability during the gait cycle. The lesser MPJs progress from subluxation to frank dislocation. Chronic dorsal dislocation of the lesser MPJs causes the primary plantarflexor stabilizers of the MPJ (interossei and lumbricles) to be elevated above the axis of rotation of the MPJ, making them ineffective at stabilization of the MPJ. The imbalance between the intrinsic and extrinsic muscles also contributes to contracture deformities at the MPJ and lesser digits.[31] These biomechanical abnormalities lead to the classic rheumatoid forefoot deformity. Patients with RA presenting with deformities of the forefoot present a difficult challenge for the podiatric surgeon. With long-standing deformity, there is a lack of tissue pliability from the digits being in a chronically contracted state. Hammer toe and claw toe deformities progress from flexible to rigid deformities. As the digit contracts and assumes a shortened position, the digital vessels also shorten. Acute digital correction can stretch or induce trauma to the digital artery, narrowing the lumen and possibly injuring the intimal layer, leading to vessel thrombosis. When vessel thrombosis is combined with narrowing of the lumen, irreversible digital ischemia may ensue, resulting in frank gangrene [6] (**Fig. 5**). In addition, reverberation from power instruments may lead to vessel spasm, further complicating the issue.[6] The podiatric surgeon must be cognizant of these possible complications and aware of the necessary measures to reverse digital vascular adverse events [6] (**Fig. 6**). The same complications may occur in any patient (namely the elderly) who undergoes acute correction of a long-standing toe deformity.

Systemic vasculitis may be a component of the progression of RA. A combination of cell-, immune-, and autoantibody-mediated inflammation of the endothelium of the blood vessel can occur. This inflammation can further increase the risk of vascular

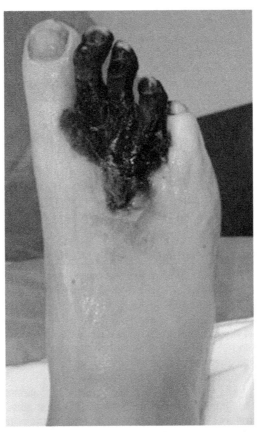

Fig. 5. Central toe and forefoot necrosis referred for treatment after attempted digital correction in a patient with diabetes.

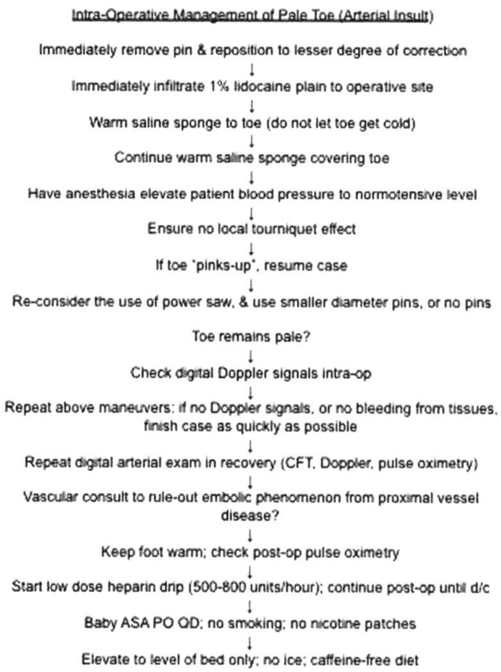

Intra-Operative Management of Pale Toe (Arterial Insult)
↓
Immediately remove pin & reposition to lesser degree of correction
↓
Immediately infiltrate 1% lidocaine plain to operative site
↓
Warm saline sponge to toe (do not let toe get cold)
↓
Continue warm saline sponge covering toe
↓
Have anesthesia elevate patient blood pressure to normotensive level
↓
Ensure no local tourniquet effect
↓
If toe "pinks-up", resume case
↓
Re-consider the use of power saw, & use smaller diameter pins, or no pins
↓
Toe remains pale?
↓
Check digital Doppler signals intra-op
↓
Repeat above maneuvers: if no Doppler signals, or no bleeding from tissues, finish case as quickly as possible
↓
Repeat digital arterial exam in recovery (CFT, Doppler, pulse oximetry)
↓
Vascular consult to rule-out embolic phenomenon from proximal vessel disease?
↓
Keep foot warm; check post-op pulse oximetry
↓
Start low dose heparin drip (500-800 units/hour); continue post-op until d/c
↓
Baby ASA PO QD; no smoking; no nicotine patches
↓
Elevate to level of bed only; no ice; caffeine-free diet

Fig. 6. Management of the acutely embarrassed toe. *From* Bibbo C. Wound healing complications and infection following surgery for rheumatoid arthritis. Foot Ankle Clin 2007;12:518; with permission.

compromise during digital surgery in the patient with RA. Proper preoperative vascular evaluation is necessary if there is any evidence suggesting arterial insufficiency. The vascular examination should begin with palpation of the dorsalis pedis and posterior tibial arteries, as well as capillary refill time of all digits. Inability to palpate pedal pulses and sluggish capillary refill is an indication to proceed with noninvasive vascular blood flow studies. The authors recommend performing segmental limb pressure measurements in addition to the ankle brachial index, because this can help determine the level at which the arterial disease is located. The generalized rule is that, if pressure measurements decrease by more than 20 mm Hg from continuous segments, disease is located in the more proximal segment. Transcutaneous oxygen pressure (TcPo$_2$) and skin perfusion pressure (SPP) measurements can also be used as indications of the status of the microcirculation and healing potential (**Table 1**).[32] In a study by Adera and colleagues[33] documenting the results of 62 limbs undergoing amputation, an SPP greater than 30 mm Hg had a positive predictive value of healing. These noninvasive vascular studies become exponentially important if the patient with RA is also diabetic or a smoker. Preoperative evaluation of vascular status is critical not only in the patient with RA, but in all surgical patients to minimize vascular compromise and possible postoperative complications.

Avascular Necrosis of the Lesser Metatarsals Following Surgery

Many surgical procedures have been described to help alleviate symptoms associated with lesser metatarsalgia, ranging from soft-tissue balancing procedures to numerous distal metatarsal osteotomies. Avascular necrosis of the lesser metatarsals

Table 1
TcPo$_2$ as a predictor of healing potential

Healing Potential	TcPo$_2$ (mm Hg)
High	>30
Intermediate	20–29
Low	<20

Data from Sage RA, Pinzur M, Stuck R, et al. Amputations and rehabilitation of the diabetic foot. In: Veves A, Giurini JM, LoGerfo FW, editors. The diabetic foot. 2nd edition. Totowa (NJ): Humana Press: 2006, p. 366–7.

following forefoot surgery and delayed or nonunion of osteotomy sites are known complications associated with these procedures. Extensive research has evaluated the risk of postoperative avascular necrosis of the first metatarsal head following osteotomy or soft-tissue release, with limited research discussing its prevalence in lesser metatarsal procedures. This difference is likely in part to the result of the significantly greater number of first metatarsal procedures being performed compared with lesser metatarsal procedures, and in part because of the paucity of literature describing the anatomic vascular supply of the lesser metatarsals.

In a cadaveric study described by Petersen and colleagues[34] in 2002, the arterial supply of the lesser metatarsals was evaluated and discussed. The lesser metatarsal heads have 2 primary sources of blood supply. The dorsalis pedis artery gives off branches supplying the dorsal aspect of the metatarsals, and the posterior tibial artery branches help to supply the plantar aspect. These branches are the dorsal and plantar metatarsal arteries, which have anastamoses with each other surrounding the lesser metatarsal heads. This network of arteries not only provides excellent extraosseous blood supply but also contributes small nutrient vessels that penetrate the cortex near the metatarsal neck to provide blood to subchondral bone. Of particular importance is the exact location of this penetration through the cortex at approximately 2 to 7 mm proximal to the MPJ articular surface, which lies immediately adjacent to capsular and ligamentous insertions such as the collateral ligaments.[34] Care must be taken by the surgeon to minimize soft-tissue stripping in the area of these collateral ligaments when performing a distal metatarsal osteotomy. Petersen and colleagues[34] described a safe distance of 3 to 4 mm from their insertions to reduce chances of vascular compromise. In a further evaluation of the intraosseous blood supply to the metatarsal heads, Petersen and colleagues[34] reported that these nutrient arteries are end arteries, unlike nutrient arteries to the diaphyseal region, which have a vast network of anastomoses. Therefore, the blood supply of the metatarsal head should be considered fragile, and any disruption increases the patient's chance of developing postoperative avascular necrosis.

The surgeon must also always be cognizant of sound surgical technique when performing an osteotomy of the lesser metatarsals. In a study by Eriksson[35] exposure to temperatures of 42 degrees Celsius can cause vascular injury and temperatures of 50 degrees Celsius for 1 minute can cause widespread tissue injury in bone.[36] Although the heat generated from power instrumentation alone is not likely to be the sole reason for avascular necrosis following osteotomy, it may contribute to the development of this complication. The authors believe that, when power instrumentation is used to create an osteotomy, application of irrigation at the time of the cut will decrease the amount of heat produced and minimize the chance of this factor playing a role in vascular compromise. Wachter and Stoll[37] reported that a steady increase in temperature at the bone-saw interface was noted on a constant application of pressure by the saw blade. Application of variable pressure and movement of the saw blade across the osteotomy site also helps decrease the amount of generated heat. To minimize the risk of thermal necrosis, osteotomes are preferred by some surgeons.

Many underlying conditions have been proposed as potential sources or risk factors for osteonecrosis. These conditions include hemoglobinopathies such as sickle cell disease, corticosteroid therapy, Cushing disease, alcohol use, tobacco abuse, pregnancy, renal disease, inflammatory bowel disease, and gout.[36,38] Proposed mechanisms for avascular necrosis secondary to these conditions include a primary interruption of blood supply to the affected bone or an increased intramedullary pressure, causing occlusion of the venous network and infarction of bone cells.[36,39] Griffith and colleagues[40] reported a correlation between cumulative prednisolone-equivalent dose and risk of osteonecrosis, showing a risk of 0.6% for patients taking a dose less than 3 g and 13% for those receiving a dose greater than 3 g. Chronic alcohol use has also been found to be an important risk factor for avascular necrosis. Studies performed by Hirota and colleagues[38] and Matsuo and colleagues[41] found a clear and significant dose-response relationship between the amount of alcohol in milliliters consumed per week and the risk of developing avascular necrosis. Both studies also found a direct relationship between risk of avascular necrosis and patients who are current smokers and have smoked for greater than 20 pack years. It has also been proposed that corticosteroids may direct bone marrow stromal cells away from the osteoblastic pathway and into the adipocytic pathway, increasing the risk for avascular necrosis.[39,42–44]

The importance of obtaining a thorough medical history before surgery cannot be overlooked. Having an understanding of significant comorbidities that may increase the risk of avascular necrosis in lesser metatarsal surgery allows the surgeon to develop a safer and more appropriate treatment plan for the patient. Counseling on the effects of alcohol use and cigarette abuse on bone healing and possible complications that may arise must be discussed in detail with the patient. The physician should have an organized and strict protocol for ceasing use of these substances in the preoperative period to minimize the risk of vascular and bone healing complications.

Treatment of postoperative avascular necrosis of the metatarsal head should begin immediately on recognition. Bone resorption in the subchondral region causes a weakening of the underlying support structure for the articular surface, leading to collapse of the subchondral bone plate and its associated articular cartilage on weight bearing.[36] Immediate postoperative non–weight bearing or offloading of this area is crucial to early treatment of this complication. The site must be protected to prevent metatarsal head collapse and early degenerative joint disease.[45] Operative management entails procedures designed to alter the pathophysiology of the disease process, restore articular congruity, and address degenerative changes to the metatarsal head. Often used in cases of avascular necrosis of the femoral head, core decompression is designed to decrease intraosseous pressure of the metatarsal, as well as promote revascularization before structural changes at the joint surface.[46] Core decompression has been performed with good results in bones of the foot including the talus and the lesser metatarsals. In a case report by Dolce and colleagues,[47] core decompression of metatarsal heads 2 and 3 with use of a 1.1 mm Kirschner wire relieved symptoms associated with avascular necrosis. In early stages of avascular necrosis, reports of perichondral grafting with application of cancellous bone graft into a dorsal wedge made at the epiphysis have shown favorable results. The idea behind this procedure is to attempt formation of a new arterial network across the epiphyseal plate to help provide blood to the epiphysis. In a retrospective study by Helal and Gibb,[48] 9 patients in early stages of avascular necrosis underwent perichondral grafting procedures, with resolution of symptoms and improved radiographic findings noted in 8 of the 9 patients in the follow-up period ranging from 3 to 9 years after the operations. In more advanced cases of bone and articular derangement, open joint debridement may be required, which involves excision of synovitic tissue, loose bodies or exostoses, and any areas of cartilage denution. Additional stability may be achieved by means of Kirschner wire stabilization across the MPJ or short leg cast application in the postoperative period to improve the chance of successful outcome with this procedure.[41]

Floating Toe Deformity After Central Metatarsal Osteotomy and the Flail Forefoot

Central metatarsalgia is most commonly secondary to a biomechanical or structural cause. Multiple anatomic situations can lead to metatarsalgia, such as long metatarsal, plantarflexed metatarsal, or abnormal metatarsal parabola. In addition, central metatarsalgia is commonly associated with hammer digit syndrome. Hammer digit syndrome often leads to a retrograde buckling of the MPJ complex and increased plantar pressure on the associated metatarsal head.[49,50] Numerous surgical options are available to treat this deformity, such as distal V osteotomy, resection arthroplasty, plantar condylectomy, and Weil osteotomy.[51–54] Distal metatarsal osteotomies are commonly performed with digital procedures to correct the associated hammer toe deformity and metatarsalgia. The Weil procedure has been popularized because of its simplicity, ease of fixation, and relative stability. The Weil osteotomy is an oblique cut in the metatarsal neck/shaft that is parallel to the weight-bearing surface, resulting in axial decompression of the MPJ, rather than plantarflexion of the associated metatarsal head.[49] Toe drift at the level of the MPJ can also be treated with an angular Weil osteotomy in combination with tendon transfers, Kirschner wire fixation, or possibly syndactylization. The Weil osteotomy can potentially lead to a postoperative floating toe deformity.[50,52,53] A floating toe deformity can be defined as a lack of digital purchase during the stance phase of gait.[50]

Multiple theories have been suggested in the literature as to the possible causes of the postoperative floating toe. It has been suggested that the Weil osteotomy changes the center of rotation of the MPJ axis to become more proximal and plantar. This change causes the intrinsic muscles that stabilize the digit in plantarflexion to pass dorsal to the MPJ axis and act as dorsiflexors to the associated digit.[52,55] Others believe that, by shortening the associated metatarsal, the flexor and extensor tendons passing dorsal and plantar to the associated MPJ are lengthened, disrupting their physiologic tension. This condition results in instability at the level of the MPJ, resulting in a possible floating toe deformity.[50] Other suggestions include postoperative scar contracture that may contribute to dorsal contracture of the associated digit.[50] Appropriate skin incisions can decrease the risk of scar contractures. Incisions that course longitudinally over flexion or extension joints, such as the MPJ, should be performed in a curvilinear fashion to prevent this scar contracture formation. In addition, incisions should be made parallel to the relaxed skin tension lines (RSTLs) whenever possible to minimize the tension on the incision. Incisions placed perpendicular to the RSTLs increase the tension on the wound edges, causing excessive collagen deposition and formation of hypertrophic scars or keloids. Proper surgical planning and incision placement can minimize the risk of scar contracture contributing to a floating toe deformity. Many previous studies have attempted to quantify the risk of floating toe deformity following the Weil osteotomy. In 2004, Migues and colleagues[52] found the incident rate of floating toe in 70 Weil osteotomy procedures to be 28.5%, with values approaching 50% when performed in conjunction with digital correction. Another study by Vandeputte and colleagues[56] demonstrated a 15% occurrence rate of floating toe (**Table 2**). Thus, in an effort to minimize the risk of osteotomy-related complications, it has been recommended to perform adjunctive procedures to the Weil osteotomy. Hofstaetter and colleagues[51] recommend performing an extensor tendon lengthening, removing a 2-mm slice of bone from the osteotomy site (elevating the center of rotation of the MPJ), and Kirschner wire stabilization of the digit in 5 degrees plantarflexion during postoperative healing. However, improperly sized Kirschner wires used for postoperative digital splinting can lead to digital malrotation. This potential complication can be avoided by using adequately sized Kirschner wires or double pinning the digit. Bennett and McLeod[57] recommend a modification of the Weil osteotomy that involves a preoperatively determined shortening of the metatarsal. Performing a girdlestone procedure, or flexor-to-extensor transfer at the level of the proximal phalanx of the involved digit, can help postoperative plantar purchase of the digit. Flexor-to-extensor transfers have been documented to cause stiff digits after operations as well as interdigital irritation caused by tendon bulk (**Fig. 7**). The senior author does not routinely use this procedure for this reason, and treatment may require takedown of the digital tendon transfer. However, the lead author prefers performing an arthroplasty rather than a girdlestone procedure or interphalangeal joint (IPJ) fusion for digital stabilization. Correction of digital malalignment status after IPJ arthroplasty is easier to manage than malunion or malposition of a failed attempt at an IPJ fusion (**Figs. 8 and 9**).

When performing digital procedures for the correction of digital contracture or floating toe deformity, it is not indicated to resect the base of the proximal phalanx of the digit. This resection can destabilize the digit through disruption of the attachments of intrinsic musculature, resulting in a multiple-level deformity secondary to combined mechanical imbalance of the intrinsic and extrinsic musculotendinous units. Arthroplasty of the IPJ spares more bone and minimizes the risk of a postoperative shortened digit. If there is an indication for resection of the base of the proximal phalanx, a concomitant syndactylization procedure should be performed to help stabilize the digit (**Fig. 10**). Proper preoperative planning and evaluation of the patient helps to minimize complications. All patients presenting for forefoot surgery must be preoperatively evaluated with a minimum of 2 radiographic weight-bearing views. The patient should also be examined through a gait analysis as well as non–weight bearing and weight-bearing positions in order to properly evaluate the dynamic effects of the intrinsic and extrinsic muscles on the lesser rays. A thorough preoperative assessment of the patient, as well as adequate intraoperative clinical assessment, helps to expose multiplane digital deformities that may require a combination of bone and soft-tissue procedures such as dermoplasty. A comprehensive understanding of the deformity being treated and proper surgical planning can avoid such complications.

Table 2
Incidence of floating toe deformity following lesser metatarsal osteotomy

Reference	Incidence (%)
Vandeputte et al, 2000[56]	15
Tollafield, 2001[70]	22
O'Kane and Kilmartin, 2002[71]	20
Migues et al, 2004[52]	28.5 overall 50 with PIPJ arthrodesis
Beech et al, 2005[72]	33

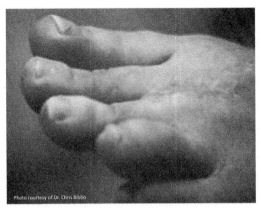

Fig. 7. Curved, stiff, swollen toes 2 and 3 after flexor-to-extensor transfers; imbalance with toes 4/5 is also present.

Complications of Distraction Osteogenesis in Brachymetatarsia

Brachymetatarsia is an abnormal shortening of one of the metatarsal bones in comparison with uninvolved metatarsals (most commonly the fourth metatarsal), with a reported incidence of 0.02% to 0.05% among the general population.[58] Several syndromes may exhibit brachymetatarsia, but the most commonly encountered is the idiopathic variety (**Box 2**). The exact molecular cause of brachymetatarsia is still

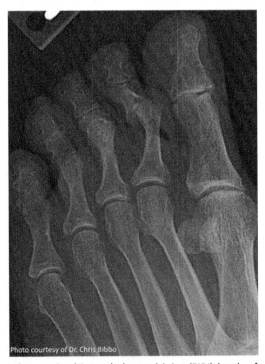

Fig. 8. Deformity at the proximal interphalangeal joint (PIPJ) level referred after arthrodesis. Deformity is caused by inadequate fixation technique.

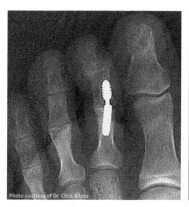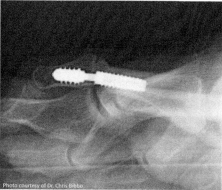

Fig. 9. Patient referred for second toe pain and metatarsalgia. Seemingly adequate PIPJ #2 arthrodesis on anteroposterior view (*left panel*). Clinical examination and lateral view (*right panel*) reveals toe elevatus and mallet deformity, both of which may be difficult to salvage.

uncertain, but errors of encoded critical growth factors involved in limb development may ultimately be implicated.

Distraction osteogenesis is a commonly used method for surgical correction of this deformity and has been reported to have advantages compared with single-stage lengthening with bone graft application. The advantages include lack of need for bone grafting, ability to bear weight earlier, and simultaneous lengthening of the

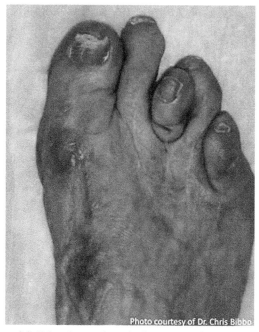

Fig. 10. Appearance of flail forefoot referred after overexuberant bone resection at inappropriate joint levels. Correction is difficult and may require multiple digital osteotomies, tendon balancing, and syndactylizations.

Box 2
Potential causes of brachymetatarsia

Congenital Down syndrome

Iatrogenic Turner syndrome

Posttraumatic Apert syndrome

Down syndrome pseudohypoparathyroidism

Multiple epiphyseal dysplasia

soft-tissue and neurovascular structures, which minimizes neurovascular insult and maximizes potential lengthening of the metatarsal. However, this method of correction has shown multiple postoperative complications including limitation of motion at the MPJ, pin-tract infections, angulation of the metatarsal, callus fracture, flexion deformities of the digits, neurovascular injury, and instability with subluxation or frank dislocation at the MPJ level.[59,60] Other potential complications of distraction osteogenesis include osteonecrosis and plantar sulcus maceration.[61]

Some of the more common complications associated with lengthening by callus distraction include postoperative joint stiffness and instability with subluxation of the MPJ. Gradual lengthening of bone directly results in resistance from tendons and other soft-tissue attachments such as the transverse metatarsal ligament and extensor and flexor sheaths.[62] In 1999, Masada and colleagues[63] reported that these complications could be reduced by limiting metatarsal lengthening to no more than 40% of its original length. In a study performed by Wada and colleagues,[62] 10 of 12 metatarsal lengthening procedures produced some degree of joint stiffness, narrowing of joint space, and plantar subluxation of the MPJ during distraction. In 11 of the 12 patients in this study, the metatarsal lengthening exceeded 40% of the original metatarsal length, with 1 patient exceeding 61% of the original length as a result of inadequate follow-up. In order to help prevent postoperative joint subluxation in patients requiring greater metatarsal lengthening, it has been recommended to apply temporary Kirschner wire stabilization across the MPJ to help hold the digit in a plantarflexed position, or perform an extensor tendon lengthening.[64,65] In a case report by Kawashima and colleagues,[66] joint stiffness and subluxation were observed in all 4 patients undergoing callus distraction.[62] Rate of distraction in these cases measured 0.7 mm/d, and it was concluded by the author that this rate of distraction was adequate for bone formation, but too fast for soft-tissue elongation.[66] Varying opinions regarding appropriate rate of distraction for these procedures can be found in the literature, and range from 0.5 mm/d to 1 mm/d. Choi and colleagues[67] reported good results with minimal complications distracting at a rate of 0.5 mm/d. Another study by Oh and colleagues[64] reviewed the results of 47 metatarsal lengthening procedures and the results included 13 cases of MPJ stiffness and 6 cases of joint subluxation when distracting at a rate of 0.5 mm/d (**Table 3**). Cases of distal metatarsal angulation following distraction have been reported. In a study of 47 distraction procedures by Oh and colleagues,[64] the greatest complication was varus angulation of the distal metatarsal fragment, reporting greater than 5 degrees of angulation in 17 cases. The most common causes for this complication include callus fracture, trauma, or iatrogenic causes.

An advantage of callus distraction compared with bony block interposition is the ability of the patient to weight bear immediately after the operation. The treating physician must be cognizant of the patient's normal lifestyle and activity level, and should discuss appropriate limitations during the postoperative course with the patient to

Table 3
Rate of distraction and incidence of lesser MPJ stiffness in surgical correction of brachymetatarsia

Study	Rate of Distraction (mm/d)	Joint Stiffness (%)
Kawishima et al,[66] 1994	0.7	100 (4/4)
Masada et al,[63] 1999	0.5	33.3 (2/6)
Choi et al,[67] 1999	0.5	11.1 (1/9)
Oh et al,[64] 2003	0.5	27.6 (13/47)
Wada et al,[62] 2004	0.7	83.3 (10/12)

avoid possible traumatic complications. If callus fracture does occur, appropriate reduction or corrective osteotomies may be necessary to aid in stabilization of the metatarsal as well as minimize gross angulation.[59] Although technically more difficult to make the corticotomy or osteotomy at the level of the metaphysis without producing greater vascular compromise secondary to a firmly attached periosteum at this level, osteotomy placement in metaphyseal bone limits the risk of callus fracture caused by increased anatomic vascularity and larger bone diameter compared with diaphyseal bone.[65] Appropriate positioning and application of the external fixator device and its pins is also imperative to prevent angulation in any abnormal plane. Pins should be placed perpendicular to the long axis of the metatarsal shaft to ensure that the external fixator is perfectly parallel to the underlying metatarsal.[65] Even mild deviation from this may result in abnormal forces on distraction, especially in the frontal and transverse planes. If excessive, these forces may also increase the risk of callus fracture. If osteotomy is performed rather than corticotomy, care must be taken that the cut be perpendicular to the weight-bearing axis of the foot.[65] This helps minimize any abnormal angulation in the sagittal plane. Future studies with the use of multiplanar minirail fixators in this type of procedure may help show decreased complication rates associated with angulation.

A flexion deformity of the associated digit can be seen in the single-stage bone inter-position procedure as well as with distraction osteogenesis. This deformity is more likely to occur in a plantarward direction, but dorsal contracture of the proximal phalanx on the head of the metatarsal has also been reported. On lengthening of the metatarsal, increased tension is placed on the flexor and extensor tendons and joint capsule structures, altering the windlass mechanism and causing increased contracture of the digit as well as the plantar capsule. Postdistraction procedures may be required to alleviate this tension, including Z-lengthening or tenotomy of the long and short flexor tendons at the level of the MPJ, lengthening or tenotomy of the long and short extensor tendons, or plantar capsulotomy if thickening of the plantar capsule is appreciated.[59,68] A delicate balance between tension on the flexor and extensor structures must be appreciated intraoperatively to obtain a more natural postoperative toe posture.[68] Kim and colleagues[68] reported an association between the amount of metatarsal lengthening and the risk of flexion deformity, relating an increased risk of this complication in metatarsals lengthened more than 40% of their original length. Oh and colleagues[64] had better results with postoperative joint contracture in children compared with adults, likely secondary to soft-tissue laxity. They recommended the procedure be performed between the ages of 14 and 21 years, after fusion of the metatarsal epiphyses is complete.

Although gradual lengthening of the metatarsal has been shown to decrease the risk of neurovascular injury compared with acute lengthening, this potential complication must still be taken seriously. Nerve complications may include neuro-praxia, neuritis, neurolysis, neuroma or nerve entrapment, and complex regional pain syndrome. Evaluating the onset time of nerve-related symptoms following this procedure can guide the surgeon to a better understanding of the underlying cause. In patients with parasthesias or hyperesthesia in the early postoperative period before initiation of lengthening, possible causes include poor surgical technique or surgical trauma, including injury from wires and pins or other surgical instrumentation necessary to perform the osteotomy or corticotomy. This hyperesthesia usually soon turns to hypoesthesia.[69] A different mechanism of nerve injury has been described for those patients with similar symptoms during the period of gradual lengthening. Safe pin placement for the external fixation device is a crucial component of this procedure. A pin located in close proximity to a nerve may become a tether to the nerve as gradual traction is applied, leading to nerve irritation and possible compromise.[69] To minimize these risks, the surgeon must have a firm understanding of neurovascular anatomy and must develop a sound surgical plan in the preoperative period. Nerve entrapment during or following gradual lengthening is also a potential complication. As the nerve and soft-tissue structures gradually stretch, tension is not only placed on the nerve itself, but formation of surrounding scar tissue can also impart compression on the nerve. Slowing the rate of lengthening may be enough to allow tension on the nerve to subside, although future consideration of nerve decompression surgery may be required in debilitating cases.

Appropriate preoperative patient education is as important as sound surgical planning and technique. The physician should understand the patient's postoperative goals and desires, and realistic goals and outcomes should be discussed in detail with the patient. The patient needs to be informed of the possible complications associated with this procedure as well as the potential necessity for adjunctive procedures to help minimize these complications or future procedures to help treat a complication.

REFERENCES

1. Chaudry SB, Liporace FA, Gandhi A, et al. Complications of ankle fracture in patients with diabetes. J Am Acad Orthop Surg 2008;16:159–70.
2. Bibbo C, Patel DV. Diabetic neuropathy. Foot Ankle Clin 2006;11:753–74.
3. Loder RT. The influence of diabetes mellitus on the healing of closed fractures. Clin Orthop Relat Res 1988;232:210–6.
4. Lodder MC, de Jong Z, Kostense PJ, et al. Bone mineral density in patients with rheumatoid arthritis: relation between disease severity and low bone mineral density. Ann Rheum Dis 2004;63(12):1576–80.
5. Bibbo C, Anderson RB, Davis WH, et al. The influence of rheumatoid chemotherapy, age, and presence of rheumatoid nodules on postoperative complications in rheumatoid foot and ankle surgery: analysis of 725 procedures in 104 patients. Foot Ankle Int 2003;24(1):1–5.
6. Bibbo C. Wound healing complications and infection following surgery for rheumatoid arthritis. Foot Ankle Clin 2007;12:509–24.
7. Abu-Rumman P, Armstrong DG, Nixon BP. Use of clinical laboratory parameters to evaluate wound healing potential in diabetes mellitus. J Am Podiatr Med Assoc 2002;92(1):38–47.
8. Konstantinides NN, Lehmann S. The impact of nutrition on wound healing. Crit Care Nurse 1993;13:25.

9. Bibbo C, Patel DV, Gehrmann RM, et al. Chlorhexidine provides superior skin decontamination in foot and ankle surgery. Clin Orthop 2005;438:204–8.
10. Brown WC, Hahn DB. Frostbite of the feet after cryotherapy: a report of two cases. J Foot Ankle Surg 2009;48(5):577–80.
11. Deodhar AK, Rana RE. Surgical physiology of wound healing: a review. J Postgrad Med 1997;43(2):52–6.
12. Bernard L, Lubbeke A, Stern R, et al. Value of preoperative investigations in diagnosing prosthetic joint infection: retrospective study and review of the literature review. Scand J Infect Dis 2004;36:410–6.
13. Ishikawa SN, Murphy GA, Richardson EG. The effect of smoking on hindfoot fusions. Foot Ankle Int 2002;23:996–8.
14. Krannitz KW, Fong HW, Fallat LM, et al. The effect of cigarette smoking on radiographic bone healing after elective foot surgery. J Foot Ankle Surg 2009;48(5):525–7.
15. Gong Z, Wezeman FH. Inhibitory effect of alcohol on osteogenic differentiation in human bone marrow-derived mesenchymal stem cells. Alcohol Clin Exp Res 2004;28(3):468–79.
16. Bibbo C, Anderson RB, Davis WH. Complications of midfoot and hindfoot arthrodesis. Clin Orthop 2001;391:45–58.
17. Bibbo C, Patel DV, Haskell MD. Recombinant bone morphogenetic protein-2 (rhBMP-2) in high-risk ankle and hindfoot fusions. Foot Ankle Int 2009;30: 597–603.
18. Bibbo C, Bono CM, Lin SS. Union rates using autologous platelet concentrate alone and with bone graft in high-risk foot and ankle surgery patients. J Surg Orthop Adv 2005;14:17–22.
19. Liporace FA, Bibbo C, Azid V, et al. Bioadjuncts for complex ankle and hindfoot reconstruction. Foot Ankle Clin 2007;12:75–106.
20. Chen D, Zhao M, Mundy GR. Bone morphogenetic proteins. Growth Factors 2004;22:233–41.
21. Gandi A, Bibbo C, Pinzur M, et al. The role of platelet-rich plasma in foot and ankle surgery. Foot Ankle Clin 2005;10:621–37.
22. Smith WR, Ziran BH, Anglen JO, et al. Locking plates: tips and tricks. J Bone Joint Surg Am 2007;89:2298–307.
23. Hallab N, Merritt K, Jacobs JJ. Metal sensitivity in patients with orthopaedic implants. J Bone Joint Surg Am 2001;83(3):428–36.
24. Joseph WS. Surgical infections and prophylaxis. In: Handbook of lower extremity infections. 2nd edition. St Louis (MO): Elsevier; 2003. p. 130–42.
25. Hargreaves DG, Drew SJ, Eckersley R. Kirschner wire pin tract infection rates: a randomized controlled trial between percutaneous and buried wires. J Hand Surg Br 2004;29(4):374–6.
26. Steckelberg J, Osmon D. Prosthetic joint infections. In: Waldvogel F, Bisno A, editors. Infections associated with indwelling medical devices. 3rd edition. Washington, DC: American Society for Microbiology Press; 2000.
27. Richter D, Hahn MP, Laun RA, et al. Arthrodesis of the infected ankle and subtalar joint: technique, indications, and results of 45 consecutive cases. J Trauma 1999; 47(6):1072–8.
28. Hoyle BD, Jass J, Costerton W. The biofilm glycocalyx as a resistant factor. J Antimicrob Chemother 1990;26:1–6.
29. Worsing RA Jr, Engber WD, Lange TA. Reactive synovitis from particulate silastic. J Bone Joint Surg Am 1982;64(4):581–5.
30. Michelson J, Easley M, Wigley FM, et al. Foot and ankle problems in rheumatoid arthritis. Foot Ankle Int 1994;15(11):608–13.

31. Jeng C, Campbell J. Current concepts review: the rheumatoid forefoot. Foot Ankle Int 2008;29(9):959–68.
32. Sage RA, Pinzur M, Stuck R, et al. Amputations and rehabilitation of the diabetic foot. In: Veves A, Giurini JM, LoGerfo FW, editors. The diabetic foot. 2nd edition. Totowa (NJ): Humana Press; 2006. p. 366–7.
33. Adera HM, James K, Castronuovo JJ, et al. Prediction of amputation wound healing with skin perfusion pressure. J Vasc Surg 1995;21(5):823–9.
34. Petersen WJ, Lankes JM, Paulsen F, et al. The arterial supply of the lesser metatarsal heads: a vascular injection study in human cadavers. Foot Ankle Int 2002; 23(6):491–5.
35. Eriksson R. Heat-induced bone tissue injury: an in vivo investigation of heat tolerance of bone tissue and temperature rise in drilling of cortical bone [dissertation]. University of Gothenburg, Sweden, 1984.
36. Banks A. Avascular necrosis of the first metatarsal head: a different perspective. J Am Podiatr Med Assoc 1999;89(9):441–53.
37. Wachter R, Stoll P. Increase of temperature during osteotomy: in vitro and in vivo investigations. Int J Oral Maxillofac Surg 1991;20:245.
38. Hirota Y, Hirohata T, Fukuda K, et al. Association of alcohol intake, cigarette smoking, and occupational status with the risk of idiopathic osteonecrosis of the femoral head. Am J Epidemiol 1993;137:530–8.
39. Mont M, Jones L, Hungerford D. Nontraumatic osteonecrosis of the femoral head: ten years later. J Bone Joint Surg Am 2006;88:1117–32.
40. Griffith JF, Antonio GE, Kumta SM, et al. Osteonecrosis of hip and knee in patients with severe acute respiratory syndrome treated with steroids. Radiology 2005; 235:168–75.
41. Matsuo K, Hirohata T, Sugioka Y, et al. Influence of alcohol intake, cigarette smoking, and occupational status on idiopathic osteonecrosis of the femoral head. Clin Orthop Relat Res 1988;234:115–23.
42. Wang GJ, Cui Q. The pathogenesis of steroid-induced osteonecrosis and the effect of lipid-clearing agents on this mechanism. In: Urbaniak JR, Jones JP, editors. Osteonecrosis: etiology, diagnosis, and treatment. Rosemont (IL): American Academy of Orthopaedic Surgeons; 1997. p. 159–66.
43. Wang GJ, Cui Q, Balian G. The pathogenesis and prevention of steroid induced osteonecrosis. Clin Orthop Relat Res 2000;370:295–310.
44. Suh KT, Kim SW, Roh HL, et al. Decreased osteogenic differentiation of mesenchymal stem cells in alcohol-induced osteonecrosis. Clin Orthop Relat Res 2005;431:220–5.
45. Wallace G, Bellacosa R, Mancuso J. Avascular necrosis following distal first metatarsal osteotomies: a survey. J Foot Ankle Surg 1994;33(2):167–72.
46. Carmont M, Rees R, Bludell M. Current concepts review: Freiberg's disease. Foot Ankle Int 2009;30(2):167–76.
47. Dolce M, Osher L, McEneaney P, et al. The use of surgical core decompression as treatment for avascular necrosis of the second and third metatarsal heads. The Foot 2006;17:162–6.
48. Helal B, Gibb P. Freiberg's disease: a suggested pattern of management. Foot Ankle 1987;8:94–102.
49. Yu GV, Judge MS, Hudson JR, et al. Predislocation syndrome. Progressive subluxation/dislocation of the lesser metarsophalangeal joint. J Am Podiatr Med Assoc 2002;92(4):182–99.
50. Derner R, Meyr AJ. Complications and salvage of elective central metatarsal osteotomies. Clin Podiatr Med Surg 2009;26:23–35.

51. Hofstaetter SG, Trnka H-J, Easley ME. The Weil osteotomy for subluxated or dislocated metatarsalphalangeal joint. Tech Foot Ankle Surg 2006;5(2):126–32.
52. Migues A, Slullitel G, Bilbao F, et al. Floating-toe deformity as a complication of the Weil osteotomy. Foot Ankle Int 2004;25(9):609–13.
53. Hamilton KD, Anderson JG, Bohay DR. Current concepts in metatarsal osteotomies: a remedy for metatarsalgia. Tech Foot Ankle Surg 2009;8(2):77–84.
54. Roukis TS. Central metatarsal head-neck osteotomies: indications and operative techniques. Clin Podiatr Med Surg 2005;22:197–222.
55. Trnka HJ, Nyska M, Parks BG. Dorsiflexion contracture after the Weil osteotomy: results of cadaver study and three-dimensional analysis. Foot Ankle 2001;22:47–50.
56. Vandeputte G, Dereymaeker G, Steenwerckx A, et al. The Weil osteotomy of the lesser metatarsals: a clinical and pedobarographic follow-up study. Foot Ankle Int 2000;21(5):370–4.
57. Bennett AJ, McLeod I. An adaptation of Weil's osteotomy of the lesser metatarsal neck. J Foot Ankle Surg 2009;48(4):516–7.
58. Shim J, Park S. Treatment of brachymetatarsia by distraction osteogenesis. J Pediatr Orthop 2006;26(2):250–4.
59. Wilusz A, Van P, Pupp G. Complications associated with distraction osteogenesis for the correction of brachymetatarsia: a review of five procedures. J Am Podiatr Med Assoc 2007;97(3):189–94.
60. Lee WC, Suh JS, Moon JS, et al. Treatment of brachymetatarsia of the first and fourth ray in adults. Foot Ankle Int 2009;30(10):981–5.
61. Lee WC, Yoo JH, Moon JS. Lengthening of fourth brachymetatarsia by three different surgical techniques. J Bone Joint Surg Br 2009;91(11):1472–7.
62. Wada A, Bensahel H, Takamura K, et al. Metatarsal lengthening by callus distraction for brachymetatarsia. J Pediatr Orthop 2004;13(3):206–10.
63. Masada K, Fujita S, Fuji T, et al. Complications following metatarsal lengthening by callus distraction for brachymetatarsia. J Pediatr Orthop 1999;19(3):394–7.
64. Oh C, Sharma R, Song H, et al. Complications of distraction osteogenesis in short fourth metatarsals. J Pediatr Orthop 2003;23:484–7.
65. DeHeer P. Forefoot applications of external fixation. Clin Podiatr Med Surg 2003;20:27–44.
66. Kawashima T, Yamada A, Ueda A, et al. Treatment of brachymetatarsia by callus distraction (callotasis). Ann Plast Surg 1994;32:191–9.
67. Choi I, Chung M, Baek G, et al. Metatarsal lengthening in congenital brachymetatarsia: one-stage lengthening versus lengthening by callotasis. J Pediatr Orthop 1999;19:660–4.
68. Kim H, Lee S, Yoo C, et al. The management of brachymetatarsia. J Bone Joint Surg Br 2003;85(5):683–90.
69. Nogueira MP, Paley D, Bhave A, et al. Nerve lesions associated with limb lengthening. J Bone Joint Surg Am 2003;85(8):1502–10.
70. Tollafield DR. An audit of lesser metatarsal osteotomy by capital proximal displacement (Weil Osteotomy). British Journal of Podiatry 2001;4(1):15–9.
71. O'Kane C, Kilmartin TE. The surgical management of central metatarsalgia. Foot Ankle Int 2002;23(5):415–9.
72. Beech I, Rees S, Tagoe M. A retrospective review of the weil metatarsal osteotomy for lesser metatarsal deformities: an intermediate follow-up analysis. J Foot Ankle Surg 2005;44(5):358–64.

Surgery of the Central Rays

Catherine A. Casteel, DPM[a],*, Alex Sikorski, MD[b],
Brian E. De Yoe, DPM[c]

KEYWORDS

- Osseous central metatarsalgia • Central ray surgery
- Brachymetatarsalgia • Elongated metatarsals

Central ray surgery, although often technically simple, can lead to an inordinate number of unsatisfied patients. It is critical that the surgeon not address the foot with "tunnel vision." Successful foot and ankle surgery requires a thorough understanding of lower extremity biomechanics. Central ray surgery is most often performed for the treatment of resilient metatarsalgia. The understanding of the etiology of a patient's metatarsalgia is necessary to have a viable surgical game plan. Simply diagnosing metatarsalgia as being the result of an elongated or shortened metatarsal does not reflect a full understanding of the biomechanical importance of the first and fifth rays.[1] Conditions affecting those that can result in central ray metatarsalgia include first ray hypermobility, elevatus, hallux abducto valgus, tailor bunion, brachymetatarsia, elongated rays, effects of digital contractures, ankle equinus, pes cavus, and metatarsus adductus.

Although first and fifth ray surgeries are being covered in other articles in this issue, one must rule out these etiologies first. The purpose of this article is to address the isolated causes of osseous central metatarsalgia that are related to an elongated metatarsal and brachymetatarsalgia (**Fig. 1**). Other osseous causes include arthrosis of the central metatarsophalangeal joints (MTPJ), bone tumor or cyst, enlargement of the metatarsal head or condyles, and digital contractures; however, these causes are not covered in this article. The authors focus on surgically addressing shortened and elongated metatarsals, surgical complications, and revisional surgery (**Figs. 2 and 3**).

SHORTENING OSTEOTOMIES

There are numerous osteotomies discussed in the literature encompassing the entire anatomy of the metatarsal from proximal to distal.[2] Proximal and central metatarsal

[a] Department of Podiatry, Hunt Regional Medical Center of Greenville, 4215 Joe Ramsey Boulevard, Greenvillle, TX 75401, USA
[b] Department of Podiatry, Malteser Foot Center, Reinbach, Gerbergasse 3, Rheinbach 53359, Germany
[c] Department of Orthopedics, Metroplex Foot and Ankle, 3201 East President George Bush Highway Suite 106, Richardson, TX 75082, USA
* Corresponding author.
E-mail address: casteelc091772000@yahoo.com

Clin Podiatr Med Surg 27 (2010) 509–522
doi:10.1016/j.cpm.2010.06.002
0891-8422/10/$ – see front matter © 2010 Elsevier Inc. All rights reserved.

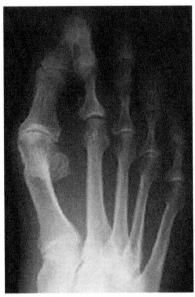

Fig. 1. AP preoperative radiograph of patient with subsecond MTPJ pain and previous bunionectomy.

osteotomies, although successful in structurally shortening a metatarsal, require a pro-longed period of non–weight bearing and are more prone to delayed or nonunion. Some distal osteotomies can result in these same issues. The authors' preferred procedure is a modified Weil-type osteotomy. The goal of the Weil osteotomy is first

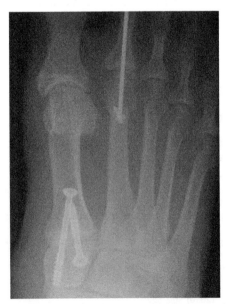

Fig. 2. AP postoperative radiograph of patient post Lapidus, second metatarsal shortening osteotomy, and hammertoe correction.

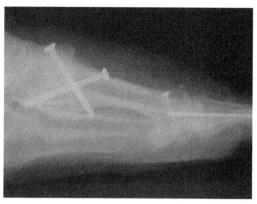

Fig. 3. Lateral postoperative radiograph showing plantigrade position of first ray.

to decompress the MTPJ and second to alter load transmission through the forefoot by shifting the plantar fragment proximal to the area of the lesion where thicker and more compliant soft tissue is still present. Although complications are few, the most commonly reported include delayed unions, dorsal adhesions at the corresponding MTPJ leading to an extensor contracture, and transfer metatarsalgia.[3–19]

The metatarsal heads have 2 arterial sources: the dorsal metatarsal arteries, which arise from the dorsalis pedis artery, and the plantar metatarsal arteries, which are branches of the posterior tibial artery. These 2 vessels typically anastomosed at 2 sites about the metatarsal heads, forming a vascular ring and provided an extensive extra-osseous arterial network around the metatarsal heads. Small arterial branches of this network run distally on the metatarsal cortex to enter the bone of the metatarsal head. The nutrient arteries traverse the cortex of the metaphysis close to the capsular and ligamentous insertions to provide multiple branches for the supply of the subchondral bone. Extensive capsular stripping during metatarsal head osteotomies results in damage to the medial and lateral head vessels;[20–22] therefore, the authors prefer to make their osteotomy at the surgical neck of the metatarsal taking great care to protect the capsular envelope of the corresponding MTPJ. By doing so, blood supply

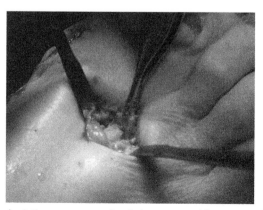

Fig. 4. Photograph depicting osseous wedge being removed from second metatarsal short-ening osteotomy.

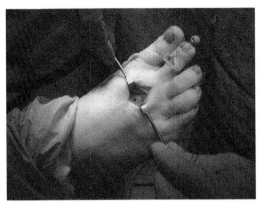

Fig. 5. Photograph depicting shortening osteotomy with fixation applied.

to the metatarsal head is protected and the chance of dorsal contracture is lessened because of a decrease in adhesions and scar tissue. The osteotomy is directed in a dorsal distal to plantar proximal fashion, then a reciprocal osteotomy is placed proximally, removing the desired amount for shortening (**Fig. 4**). Fixation is achieved with a single 2.0-mm screw directed from dorsal proximal to plantar distal taking care to not create hardware irritation plantarly (**Fig. 5**).

The procedure offers up to 5 mm of shortening with relatively minor complications noted by the authors in more than 200 procedures including no avascular necrosis or nonunions. This procedure was performed in isolated patients, which allowed immediate ambulation in a fracture walker boot for 6 weeks graduating to an athletic shoe for 4 weeks. Adjunctive procedures ultimately dictate the postoperative course.

LENGTHENING PROCEDURES

Preoperative decision making for elongating a metatarsal depends on the amount of lengthening desired. Owing to soft tissue and neurovascular constraints, osteotomies are generally limited to approximately 1 cm. Osteotomies have the benefit of fast healing, but are limited in the amount of correction available. More than 1 cm requires distraction osteogenesis with an external fixator. Distraction osteogenesis remains

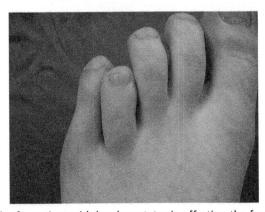

Fig. 6. Photograph of a patient with brachymetatarsia affecting the fourth metatarsal.

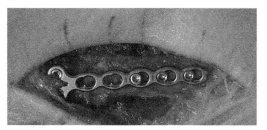

Fig. 7. Lesser metatarsal Z-lengthening with fixation applied.

an option for less than 1 cm, especially if there is significant soft tissue constraint. The benefit of distraction osteogenesis is almost unlimited lengthening; it does, however, require strict patient compliance (**Fig. 6**).

Single-stage osteotomy with interpositional bone graft, while effective in achieving length, suffers from increased complications. These include graft and host site instability leading to nonunion and malunion, and may require autogenous iliac crest graft depending on size. The authors' preferred osteotomy is the sagittal Z-lengthening, which combines both the ability to lengthen and correct angular deformity with stability. The authors perform the osteotomy at 45 degrees from dorsal medial to plantar lateral with the sagittal cut 3 times the length of lengthening desired. By doing so, rigid plate fixation can be applied to the lateral side of the metatarsal. Tibial autogenous graft is used to fill the osseous void left by distraction. The patient is kept non–weight bearing for 2 to 4 weeks and protected weight bearing for 4 weeks. Again, adjunctive procedures may dictate the postoperative course (**Fig. 7**).

Distraction osteogenesis, although technically simple, requires a compliant patient. The authors' technique is to first place the pins of the monolateral fixator and then perform the osteotomy. The most proximal pin is placed in the corresponding cuneiform or cuboid and the next pin placed in the base of the desired metatarsal. The 2 distal pins are placed approximately 2 to 3 cm distal to the osteotomy. The fixator is removed and a transverse osteotomy is performed at the proximal metaphysis. It is critical to protect and repair the periosteal envelope at the time of osteotomy to aid in healing. The fixator is then reapplied and the osteotomy is compressed for 7

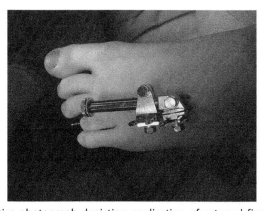

Fig. 8. Intraoperative photograph depicting application of external fixator for distraction osteogenesis of the fourth metatarsal.

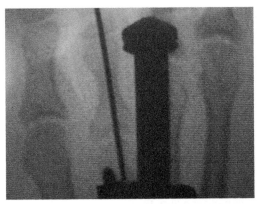

Fig. 9. AP radiograph of K-wire transfixing the fourth MTPJ and external fixator.

days. A 0.062 Kirschner wire (K-wire) is placed through the corresponding toe across the metatarsophalangeal joint at the time of surgery and left percutaneous to prevent extensor contracture during lengthening (**Fig. 8**).

After 7 days, the metatarsal is distracted at a rate of 0.5 mm twice daily spread over 12 hours until the desired lengthening has occurred. Once radiographic callous is noted, the K-wire is removed and the patient may bear weight in a surgical shoe. Once significant healing at the distraction site has occurred, the external fixator is removed. On average this time is about twice the distraction period. Bone stimulators are frequently used during this period to expedite healing. The patient then continues weight bearing in the surgical shoe for 3 to 4 weeks until there is minimal edema.

It should be noted that this procedure requires strict patient compliance and frequent surgeon follow-up. The authors do not advocate this procedure for cosmesis. This procedure, however, gives the surgeon the ability to lengthen and correct severe deformities of the metatarsal for symptomatic patients. The main complication noted by the authors is extensor contracture at the MTPJ, which is lessened by the use of a K-wire; joint stiffness is also a common complication (**Fig. 9**).

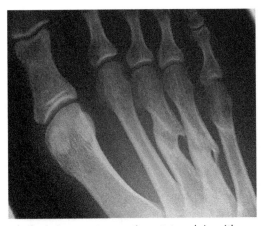

Fig. 10. AP radiograph depicting posttraumatic metatarsalgia with second MTPJ pain.

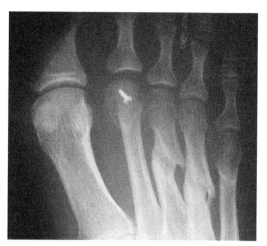

Fig. 11. AP radiograph depicting second metatarsal shortening osteotomy.

ERRORS AND FAILURES IN SURGERY OF THE CENTRAL METATARSALS

Failures in surgery of the central metatarsals are well known at least since L. Weil required modification of his osteotomy method by Barouk because of high revision rates that were reported.[23] Neglect of basic biomechanical principles and the overestimation of radiographic diagnostics are the key reasons for complications following metatarsal surgery.

Therefore, a thorough examination and documentation of foot and ankle anatomy, including the plantar aspect of the foot, is necessary before surgery on the lesser metatarsals is conducted. Callous formation of the plantar region is helpful in preoperative planning for surgery of the central metatarsals. Legal actions are often caused by poorly documented clinical accounts of the symptoms presented and/or inadequate description of the intended procedures by the surgeon.

General Error

Biomechanical misjudgment

The first ray is the primary weight carrier of the forefoot. If one isolates the mechanical ground forces applied to the metatarsal heads, the second metatarsal head is the

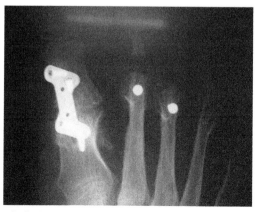

Fig. 12. AP radiograph depicting postoperative Stainsby arthroplasty.

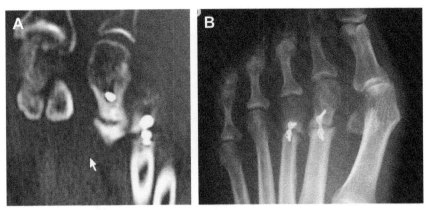

Fig. 13. (A) CT and (B) AP radiograph depicting nonunion of second and third metatarsal osteotomies.

main carrier. This delicate balance is reinforced by the rigid articulation of the second metatarsal base. Also, a disturbed alignment of the metatarsal bone and a "derailment" of the intrinsic muscles can add to a deformity of feet and toes.

On all accounts, dorsiflexion of the ankle joint must be documented. Frequently, shorted gastrocnemius/soleus muscles are the cause of a pathologic force on the forefoot. Given these facts, errors in surgical planning and well-intended but baseless procedures that quite possibly can worsen the patient's symptoms, can be avoided.

Overestimation of radiographs

Radiographs alone should not determinate the level of therapeutic intervention needed. At best, they serve to objectify the clinical findings and show axial deviations or bone deformities that may be not apparent in the physical examination.

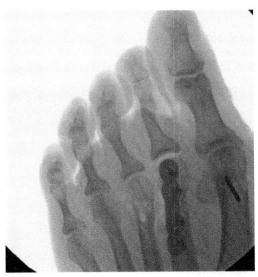

Fig. 14. AP radiograph depicting repair of nonunion with autogenous bone graft and bunionectomy.

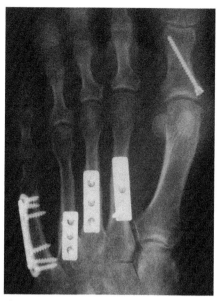

Fig. 15. AP radiograph of patient with continued subthird MTPJ pain post Akin, tailors bunionectomy, and shortening base osteotomies of second through fourth metatarsals.

Possible Solutions After Failed Metatarsal Surgery

An important prerequisite for successful revision surgery is the precise analysis of clinical complaints in regard to the biomechanics of the foot.

All options of conservative treatment methods (orthotic inserts, cushion insoles, and shoe modifications) should be exhausted before surgery is attempted.

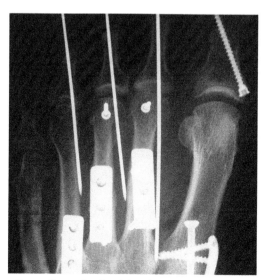

Fig. 16. AP postoperative radiograph of revisional surgery of patient in Fig. 16 with Lapidus, second and third metatarsal shortening osteotomies, and second through fourth hammertoe correction.

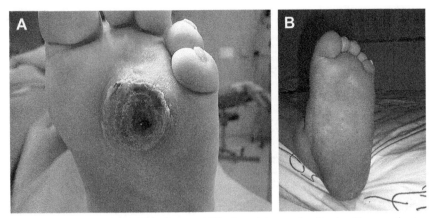

Fig. 17. "Inner amputation" (*A*) before and (*B*) after pictures of patient with cavus foot and previous lesser metatarsal surgery

Radiographic examinations, CT, and/or MRI are used to detect the initial situation and avoid poor surgical planning. Pseudoarthrosis and osteonecrosis must be ruled out in advance of surgery.

CT or MRI?

Pathologic fractures of the bone and circulatory disturbances are presented more clearly in MRI scans. The CT scan, however, is preferred when evaluation of the osseous structure before an osteotomy or athrodesis with internal fixation is still in place.

Meticulous patient education is essential, and special emphasis should be placed on the circulatory status of the toes including the documentation of preceding partial or complete loss of sensation to the digits.

Complications after Weil osteotomy

Stiffness of the MTPJ is a common complication of this shortening osteotomy. It may be caused by too small incisions initially, but also through "anatomically correct" reconstructions of the articular capsule. The authors acknowledge the deeply rooted belief that a joint capsule must always be closed after surgical intervention is still widespread.

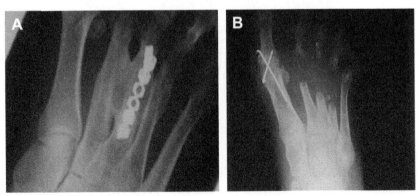

Fig. 18. AP radiograph of (*A*) pre- and (*B*) postoperative patient undergoing "inner amputation" and first MTPJ arthrodesis.

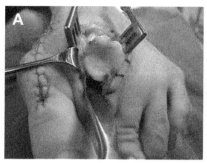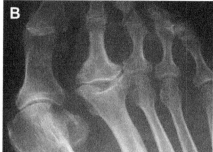

Fig. 19. (*A*) Intraoperative photograph and (*B*) preoperative radiograph of patient with avascular necrosis involving the second metatarsal.

Arthrotomy with extensive synovectomy combined with a tenolysis of the extensor tendons, is the procedure of choice. A Z-plasty of the extensor tendon eases access to the joint. A McGlamry metatarsal elevator carefully used helps to release the plantar adhesions. K-wires can be placed across the corresponding MTPJ to maintain the digit in a rectus alignment and thus preventing capsular contraction. In all cases, capsule reconstruction should be avoided. A shortening osteotomy is required when disturbed alignment of the metatarsals or dislocation of the MTPJ is noted (**Figs. 10** and **11**).

When malalignment of the MTPJ is noted and can no longer be reapproximated, one must think of the Stainsby arthroplasty: resection of the proximal phalanx base and plantar folding of the long extensor tendon.[24] This is a salvage procedure to correct severe digital deformities while preserving the metatarsal heads (**Fig. 12**).

Failures after shaft osteotomy
Painful nonunion and axis-deviations frequently make surgical revisions necessary (**Fig. 13**). Resection of the nonunion, followed by autogenous bone graft from the calcaneus or tibia with locking plate fixation is required. The use of a locking 2.7-mm plate for reconstruction in these specific cases and also for general use on fractures of the metatarsal area is highly recommended (**Figs. 14–16**).

Complications following pes cavus surgery
Forefoot surgery for a cavus foot should not primarily focus on the lesser metatarsals. Many case studies have shown this to have a high failure rate.[1,25,26]

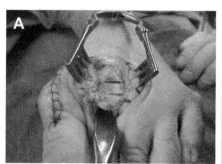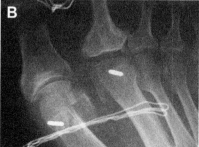

Fig. 20. (*A*) Photograph of intracapital closing-wedge osteotomy of the second metatarsal head and (*B*) AP postoperative radiograph.

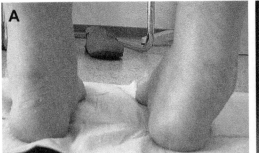
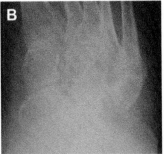

Fig. 21. (*A*) Photograph and (*B*) AP radiograph of a patient with Jones fracture of the fifth metatarsal base in a cavus foot.

In cases of remaining metatarsalgia and the correction of the "reverse buckling" by proximal interphalangeal joint arthrodesis of the toes, Z-plasty of the extensor tendons and release of MTPJ symptoms can remain. In particularly severe cases involving plantar ulcerations, a partial metatarsal resection or "inner amputation" of the central 3 rays and first MTPJ arthrodesis is the ultimate solution (**Fig. 17**). Relief is provided by diverting the anatomy and creating a 3-point weight-bearing surface of the forefoot. Accommodative insoles are mandatory in a patient's postoperative treatment (**Fig. 18**).

Complications involving osteonecrosis

Remaining metatarsalgia and stiffness of the affected MTPJ may require revision surgery. Arthrotomy with osteophyte resection and a modified intra-articular dorsal closing-wedge osteotomy is performed (**Figs. 19** and **20**).

Chondral grafting (OATS procedure) from the ipsilateral knee is a viable option if there is insufficient cartilage available plantarly. The Stainsby arthroplasty, originally a method of the rheumatic surgery, should be applied only in severe cases.

Cavus foot stress fractures

Microfractures, which are caused by mechanical overload, heal uneventfully with conservative therapy and long-term orthotic therapy. Stress fractures and

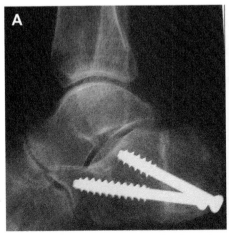
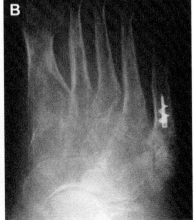

Fig. 22. (*A*) Three-year postoperative lateral and (*B*) AP radiograph of patient in Fig. 22 treated with Dwyer calcaneal osteotomy and reattachment of the peroneus brevis tendon.

pseudarthrosis at the base of the fifth metatarsal are often caused by increased pull of the peroneus brevis tendon owing to an imbalance with the posterior tibial tendon. In these cases, nonunions can result and may require open reduction with internal fixation and autogenous bone grafting. Also, a reduction of the peroneal tendon tension by Z-plasty and calcaneus valgus osteotomy is required (**Figs. 21** and **22**).

Summary of Errors and Failures in Surgery of the Central Metatarsals

Revisional surgery of the lesser metatarsals requires thorough understanding of lower extremity biomechanics. All conservative measures must be used before any surgery is undertaken. The multiple possibilities of revision surgery must be applied with detailed consideration of the underlying biomechanical function of the foot. In all cases, isolated resection of the metatarsal head should be avoided because of the possibility of transfer metatarsalgia. The Stainsby arthroplasty is a good alternative for severe cases of MTPJ dislocation. Inner amputation can be considered as a last resort when all other specific reliefs for plantar lesions have been unsuccessful.

SUMMARY

Procedures to both lengthen and shorten the central rays, although often technically simple, do not always result in satisfactory results for the patient. Establishing a normal parabola within the forefoot without establishing function of the first and fifth rays will result in suboptimal patient outcomes. Particular attention to fixation and preservation of the circulation to the central rays lessens the likelihood of delayed and nonunions. As with all foot and ankle surgeries, preoperative biomechanical analysis is critical for a good outcome.

REFERENCES

1. Viladot A. Metatarsalgia due to biomechanical alterations of the forefoot. Orthop Clin North Am 1973;4(1):165–78.
2. Baravarian B. Lesser metatarsal osteotomy. In: Chang TJ, editor. Master techniques in podiatric surgery: the foot and ankle. Philadelphia: Lippincott, Williams and Wilkins; 2005. p. 85–92.
3. Snyder J, Owen J, Wayne J, et al. Plantar pressure and load in cadaver feet after a Weil or chevron osteotomy. Foot Ankle Int 2005;26(2):158–65.
4. Beech I, Rees S, Tagoe M. A retrospective review of the Weil metatarsal osteotomy for lesser metatarsal deformities: an intermediate follow-up analysis. J Foot Ankle Surg 2005;44(5):358–64.
5. Lauf E, Weinraub GM. Asymmetric "V" osteotomy: a predictable surgical approach for chronic central metatarsalgia. J Foot Ankle Surg 1996;35(6):550–9.
6. Jimenez AL, Fishco WD. Part 3: central metatarsals. In: Banks AS, Downey MS, Martin DE, et al, editors. McGlamary's comprehensive textbook of foot and ankle surgery. Philadelphia: Lippincott, William and Wilkins; 2001. p. 322–38.
7. Yu GV, Judge MS, Hudson JR, et al. Predislocation syndrome. Progressive subluxation/dislocation of the lesser metatarsophalangeal joint. J Am Podiatr Med Assoc 2002;92(4):182–99.
8. Hacther RM, Gollier WL, Weil LS. Intractable plantar keratoses: a review of surgical corrections. J Am Podiatr Med Assoc 1978;68:377–86.
9. Trnka HJ, Muhlbauer M, Zettl R, et al. Comparison of the results of the Weil and Helal osteotomies for the treatment of metatarsalgia secondary to dislocation of the lesser metatarsophalangeal joint. Foot Ankle Int 1999;20(2):72–9.

10. Trnka HJ, Nyska M, Parks BG, et al. Dorsiflexion contracture after the Weil osteotomy: results of cadaver study and three-dimensional analysis. Foot Ankle Int 2001;22(1):47–50.
11. Migues A, Slullitel G, Bilbao F, et al. Floating-toe deformity as a complication of the Weil osteotomy. Foot Ankle Int 2004;25(9):609–13.
12. Grimes J, Coughlin M. Geometric analysis of the Weil osteotomy. Foot Ankle Int 2006;27(11):985–92.
13. Helal B, Gress M. Telescoping osteotomy for pressure metatarsalgia. J Bone Joint Surg Br 1984;66:213–7.
14. Weil L. Weil head-neck oblique osteotomy-technique and fixation. Presented at Techniques of Osteotomies of the Forefoot. Bordeaux (France), October 1994.
15. Khalafi A, Laundsman AS, Lautenschlager EP, et al. Plantar forefoot changes after second metatarsal neck osteotomy. Foot Ankle Int 2005;26(7):550–5.
16. Johnson RB III, Smith J, Daniels T. The plantar plate of the lesser toes: an anatomical study in human cadavers. Foot Ankle Int 1994;15:276–82.
17. Thompson FM, Hamilton WG. Problems of the second metatarsophalangeal joint. Orthopedics 1987;10:83–9.
18. Myerson MS, Jung HG. The role of the flexor-to-extensor transfer in correcting metatarsophalangeal joint instability of the second toe. Foot Ankle Int 2005;26: 675–9.
19. Schwartz N, Williams JE Jr, Marcinko DE. Double oblique lesser metatarsal osteotomy. J Am Podiatry Assoc 1983;73(4):218–20.
20. Roukis TS. Central metatarsal head-neck osteotomies: indications and operative techniques. Clin Podiatr Med Surg 2005;22(2):197–222.
21. Dockery GL. Evaluation and treatment of metatarsalgia and kerotic disorders. In: Myerson MS, editor. Foot and ankle disorders. Philadelphia: W.B. Saunders Company; 2000. p. 359–78.
22. Kennedy JG, Deland JT. Resolution of metatarsalgia following oblique osteotomy. Clin Orthop Relat Res 2006;453:309–13.
23. Barouk LS. Weil's metatarsal osteotomy in the treatment of metatarsalgia. Orthopade 1996;25(4):338–44.
24. Briggs PJ, Stainsby GD. Metatarsal head preservation in forefoot arthroplasty. Foot Ankle Surg 2001;7:93–101.
25. Feibel JB, Tisdel CL, Donley BG. Lesser metatarsal osteotomies. A biomechanical approach to metatarsalgia. Foot Ankle Clin 2001;6:473–89.
26. Helal B. Metatarsal osteotomy for metatarsalgia. J Bone Joint Surg Br 1975;57: 187–92.

Puncture Wounds of the Foot

Roger S. Racz, DPM[a], Crystal L. Ramanujam, DPM[b],
Thomas Zgonis, DPM, FACFAS[b],*

KEYWORDS

- Puncture wounds • Foot • Tetanus prophylaxis
- Osteomyelitis • Surgery

Puncture wounds are common injuries of the foot. Although most puncture wounds are benign, devastating complications are possible without adequate treatment. These injuries can occur in all age groups and in various circumstances. The clinical presentation of puncture wounds can often be misleading, while the complications of puncture wounds can involve a large range of manifestations including persistent pain, foreign body reactions, local cellulitis, abscess, osteomyelitis, and systemic infection. A thorough knowledge of proper clinical evaluation, diagnosis, microbiology, and both medical and surgical management of puncture wounds can prevent significant morbidity.

EPIDEMIOLOGY

Puncture wounds comprise a large number of cases presenting to emergency departments, and previous surveys have reported that these injuries occurred more often in summer and fall months owing to increased outdoor activity at this time of year.[1,2] Although people of all ages can sustain these injuries, children are frequently the victims. One study estimated that 1% of all emergency department visits by children are for pedal puncture wounds.[2] The most common culprits of puncture wounds are nails, with other metallic objects, glass, or wood less commonly implicated (**Fig. 1**).

Because not all patients seek treatment of puncture wounds, the true complication rate is unknown. Of those patients who seek medical attention, complication rates range from 2% to 10%.[3] Rates of infection depend on several factors including and not limited to the following: timing of presentation, location and depth of penetrating foreign object, environment of the injury, type of foreign object, previous treatment, and the immune status of the patient.[4–8]

[a] Great Falls Clinic, 3000 15th Avenue South, Great Falls, MT 59405, USA
[b] Division of Podiatric Medicine and Surgery, Department of Orthopaedic Surgery, The University of Texas Health Science Center at San Antonio, 7703 Floyd Curl Drive – MSC 7776, San Antonio, TX 78229, USA
* Corresponding author.
E-mail address: zgonis@uthscsa.edu

Clin Podiatr Med Surg 27 (2010) 523–534
doi:10.1016/j.cpm.2010.06.008
podiatric.theclinics.com

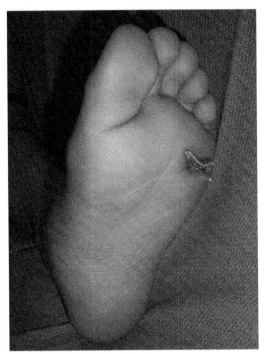

Fig. 1. Left foot of a female pediatric patient evaluated in the emergency room, who had stepped on a piece of wood 2 hours before her presentation.

CLINICAL EVALUATION

A systematic approach to assessment is essential for effective treatment. A detailed history both of the injury itself and of the patient's medical status prior to injury should be evaluated in great detail.

Time to Presentation

Patients who present after 48 hours are more likely to have complications.[7] Lavery and colleagues[5] demonstrated a significant delay in seeking treatment among diabetic patients, which led to a greater risk of osteomyelitis when compared with nondiabetic patients. Similarly, Eidelman and colleagues[9] found that delayed treatment of puncture wounds in children led to an increased risk of osteomyelitis and retained foreign body. Patients can also present to a physician long after the inciting injury because of symptoms caused by the formation of foreign body granulomas, therefore even a remote history of puncture injury can be significant. These lesions serve as local tissue chronic inflammatory reactions elicited by the retained material, and may cause severe pain or subsequent infection.[7]

Location and Depth of Injury

Puncture injuries sustained at the forefoot are more likely to cause sequelae because foreign objects may penetrate deeper at this weight-bearing surface.[7] Risk of injury to bone, tendon, or joint is also high in this area because of the close proximity of these structures to the skin. In their study of 35 patients sustaining serious plantar puncture wounds, Patzakis and colleagues[8] found 34 of these occurred in the forefoot. These investigators found a direct correlation between depth of penetration and risk of complication, and also developed a classification system dividing the plantar foot into 3 zones: (1) the metatarsal neck to the end of the toes, (2) the metatarsal neck to the distal end of the calcaneus, and (3) the body of the calcaneus. In their study, osseous involvement increased with Zone 1 and 2 puncture wounds.[8]

Environment of Injury

Puncture wounds occurring outdoors are more likely to cause contamination. Likewise, presence or absence of shoe gear or socks at the time of injury should be recorded to determine whether remnants of this footwear could have been carried into the wounds, creating an increased risk of infection.[3,10] In a study of 8 patients with deep puncture wounds from rubber-soled shoes, Chang and colleagues[4] found 3 patients with osteomyelitis of the metatarsals caused by embedded rubber fragments. The environment can also give an indication of types of pathogenic organisms involved with infection, and may shed light on the direction of therapy.[8,10]

Review of the patient's tetanus immunization history is imperative for any puncture injury.[3,11] **Table 1** provides an overview of appropriate tetanus prophylaxis.

Type of Foreign Object

As stated, nails cause the vast majority of pedal puncture wounds, yet in most cases the nails do not remain lodged in the foot and are readily identified with radiographic analysis. In a study analyzing hospital admission following nail puncture wounds, Patzakis and colleagues[8] found that the condition of the nail (clean, dirty, or rusty) did not influence the need for hospital stay. Glass may be easily retained and is difficult to identify on radiographs unless it has lead content. Montano and colleagues[12] found that puncture wounds sustained by stepping on glass had increased likelihood of retention of a foreign body. Animal hair or fur can also penetrate the soft tissues and cause formation of foreign body granulomas. Wood can splinter and is often difficult to remove completely; likewise, needles and pins break easily on contact with the foot and can be retained deep within the tissues. Imoisili and colleagues[13] reported a high occurrence of retained toothpick fragments in children sustaining pedal puncture wounds leading to infections. Selection of appropriate imaging studies for detection of foreign bodies often depends on the type of object implicated in the injury.

Table 1 CDC recommendations for tetanus prophylaxis in wound management		
History of Previous Tetanus Immunization	Clean, Minor Wounds	All Other Wounds, Including Puncture Wounds
Uncertain or fewer than 3 doses	Give vaccine	Give vaccine and TIG (250 U IM)
Three or more previous doses	No need to vaccinate Unless ≥10 years since last dose	Give vaccine If ≥5 years since last dose

Vaccine for patients 10 to 64 years old = Tdap (tetanus, reduced diphtheria, and pertussis); vaccine for patients <7 years old = DTaP (diphtheria, tetanus, acellular pertussis); vaccine for patients 7 to 9 years old and >65 years old = Td (tetanus, diphtheria).

Abbreviations: IM, intramuscular; TIG, tetanus immunoglobulin.

Previous Treatment

History pertaining to previous treatments of the wound, either by the patient or another health care professional, is important to direct further care. Overuse of topical antiseptic agents such as hydrogen peroxide may not be effective in reducing infection risk.[14] Previous antibiotic therapy, both systemic and local, can affect local bacterial flora and may induce resistance. Careful documentation of these treatments and the patient's response to them is imperative. Any attempts at removal of foreign material should also be noted regarding whether objects were removed in their entirety or if remnants may have been left in the wound; in addition, procedures attempted for removal of objects may actually force them deeper into the tissues and can alter location for later surgical approaches.

Medical History

Medical comorbidities, particularly those that compromise the immune system, may alter the clinical presentation and treatment of individuals with puncture wounds. Complete review of the patient's current medications and allergies is essential. Puncture wounds in patients with medical conditions resulting in peripheral vascular disease, neuropathy, and immunopathy can potentially cause limb- or life-threatening infections. Diabetic patients are frequently the victims of pedal puncture wounds resulting from the loss of peripheral sensation. The injury may initially go unnoticed, leading to significant delay in treatment and increased likelihood of infection.[5,6] These patients may not demonstrate the typical cardinal signs of infection and their laboratory studies may also underestimate the severity of infection.[15] Patients on immunosuppressive medications, such as those used in rheumatoid arthritis, require aggressive treatment to prevent and/or treat infections.[16] Likewise, vascular disease can limit the access of phagocytic cells and can impair the ability of antibiotics to reach the site of infection, therefore requiring alternative methods of delivery.[17]

Wound Assessment

Lack of a dramatic appearance may lead to an underestimation of wound severity. Early after injury, localized erythema and edema may or may not be present. Usual symptoms within 24 hours can include pain, ecchymosis, and swelling. The most common complication is cellulitis, which often occurs more than 24 hours following injury.[18] The level of pain may indicate infection in sensate patients. It is possible for constitutional symptoms to manifest even when the wound itself appears benign. As previously mentioned, the location and depth of the wound are extremely important in determining the extent of injury. The proximity of the puncture site to any neurovascular structure, tendon, or joint capsule should be noted. Evaluation of sensation and motor function is essential to elucidate possible damage to nerves or tendons. The skin margins should be assessed for viability because clean wound margins usually harbor fewer bacteria than irregular borders. Active drainage from the puncture wound may indicate deeper infection. Ischemic appearance of surrounding skin or the presence of necrotic tissue at the wound base may necessitate further vascular workup. A thorough inspection of the wound and surrounding areas for retained foreign material is critical. Previous reports indicate certain materials are more likely to be retained, such as rubber, which can cause "tattooing" of the skin and can elicit reactions long after the initial injury.[4,12,13] In cases of delayed treatment, the portal of entry may not be clearly visible because the wound may have already healed over the site. Patients may complain of significant pain or perception of the retained foreign body at the puncture site.[12] Septic arthritis, osteomyelitis, and/or necrotizing fasciitis can occur as major complications of pedal puncture wounds.

DIAGNOSTIC STUDIES
Radiography

Baseline plain film radiographic analysis with multiple views of the foot is recommended for all puncture wounds. These views can be useful to evaluate for retained foreign bodies, yet detection on plain films is based on the density, configuration, size, and orientation of the foreign body (**Figs. 2–4**).[19] Plain film radiography can also show evidence of osseous damage induced by the force of injury itself or by infectious processes. Underpenetrated plain radiography may facilitate detection of smaller objects. Intraoperative fluoroscopy is also useful in surgical removal. After attempts at removal of any portion of a foreign body, plain films should be taken to confirm complete retrieval. Radiography should not be used when radiation exposure is contraindicated. Soft tissue air or filling defects are sometimes apparent in plain films of nonradiopaque foreign bodies; however, advanced imaging techniques may be required for some objects containing wood, rubber, plastic, pieces of sock, or some types of glass.

Ultrasonography

For nonradiopaque foreign bodies initially missed with radiographs, ultrasonography has been reported as a reliable detection tool. Retained wooden foreign bodies are easily identified based on the leading edge of the echogenic wood resulting in marked acoustic shadowing (**Fig. 5**).[20] When compared with computed tomography (CT) and magnetic resonance imaging (MRI), ultrasonography is less expensive and more readily available. Rockett and colleagues[21] reported 100% sensitivity when using ultrasonography to rule out wooden foreign bodies in 20 patients with pedal puncture wounds. For even extremely small objects such as thorns, ultrasonography has been successful in triangulation for subsequent removal.[22] This modality can also be used intraoperatively for localization of foreign bodies but its sensitivity is operator dependent.[13,23] Shiels and colleagues[22] recommend a combination of transverse and longitudinal scanning planes to facilitate surgical removal using hemostats.

CT

CT scan is recommended for localization of metal, wood, plastic, foreign body granulomas, and collections of pus; it is also useful in detecting foreign bodies close to

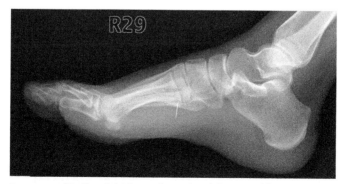

Fig. 2. Puncture wound in the right foot of a male adult, caused by stepping on a needle 1 week before his presentation. The patient had a history of diabetes and neuropathy as well as localized signs of clinical infection.

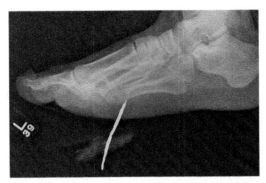

Fig. 3. Puncture wound in the right foot of a male adult, caused by stepping on a large piece of metal through the sole of a boot on a construction site 4 hours before his presentation.

bone, which may be missed with ultrasonography.[9] Three-dimensional imaging with CT is useful for surgical planning; it can also show damage to cortical bone or joint surfaces, which may not be obvious on plain film radiographs. Cadaveric studies have shown higher sensitivity of CT versus radiography in the detection of wooden foreign bodies.[24] This modality should not be used in patients for whom irradiation is prohibited. When compared with MRI, CT is faster to perform, less expensive, and more readily available.

MRI

MRI can facilitate detection of nonmetallic foreign bodies when other imaging techniques have failed. This modality should not serve as the first choice for imaging because it is not always readily accessible, is relatively expensive, and obtaining the study can be time consuming. For recalcitrant cases in which there is suspicion for infection, MRI is extremely sensitive in the identification of abscess formation and osteomyelitis. MRI studies of the foot should include T1, T2, and short-tau inversion recovery sequences with small fields of view. Foreign bodies can be visualized as signal voids within the images. Osteomyelitis is usually identified by decreased signal intensity within bone marrow on T1-weighted images and increased signal intensity on T2-weighted images. A study by Lau and colleagues[25] involving 12 patients demonstrated MRI as a reliable and cost-effective method for the diagnosis of *Pseudomonas*

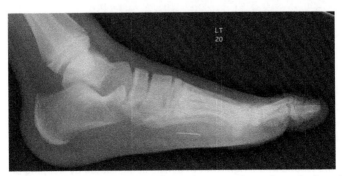

Fig. 4. Left foot of a pediatric patient with continuous pain evaluated after stepping on a needle 1 day before presentation.

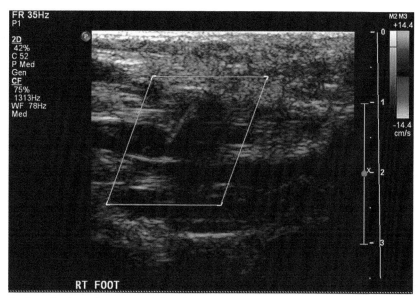

Fig. 5. A pediatric patient presented with a painful puncture wound; there was no evidence of a foreign body on plain radiographs, but ultrasonography identified a wooden splinter (1 cm echogenic linear focus).

osteomyelitis after puncture wounds. Gadolinium contrast enhancement can be used to further assess extent of involvement with soft tissue and osseous structures; however, gadolinium contrast enhancement should be used with caution in patients with kidney disease.[26]

Radionuclide Imaging

Scintigraphy can be helpful for puncture wounds of delayed presentation because it is highly sensitive for inflammatory processes such as infection, and these images show increased isotope uptake at the affected area. However, because of the lack of anatomic detail and low specificity of triple-phase technetium bone scans, these studies cannot distinguish between bone or soft tissue involvement. Furthermore, acute trauma to bone or soft tissues by the penetrating object cannot be differentiated from infectious processes such as septic arthritis and osteomyelitis; any pathologic process that creates reaction within bone leads to a positive bone scan. This point is particularly important in puncture wounds that have undergone prior exploration or debridement, because local trauma to tissues caused by dissection can elicit changes that may affect interpretation of these images. Radionuclide imaging is advantageous compared with plain film radiographs in diagnosing early osteomyelitis; technetium scans can detect osteomyelitis within 24 hours of onset, whereas radiography typically requires 10 to 14 days before changes are noted. Gelfand and Silberstein[27] used triple-phase technetium scans to confirm osteomyelitis in 16 of 19 clinically suspected cases of children with infections. In vitro labeled leukocyte scintigraphy has been reported to have higher sensitivity and specificity for diagnosing pedal osteomyelitis even among diabetic patients who commonly show misleading symptoms.[28] More recently, additional high-resolution imaging including single-photon emission, CT, and positron emission tomography have been investigated, yet data regarding these methods is limited regarding their use in distinguishing between bone and soft tissue infections of the foot.[28]

Laboratory Studies

For simple, uncomplicated puncture wounds that present for treatment in a timely fashion, there are no specific indications for laboratory tests. Complete blood cell count, erythrocyte sedimentation rate, and C-reactive protein are recommended in cases of suspected infection.[18] These tests can serve to monitor progress following surgical debridement and antibiotic therapy. Tests may be misleading in immunocompromised patients, as demonstrated by a study by Lavery and colleagues[29] that showed marked differences in values between diabetic and nondiabetic patients with infected puncture wounds. Deep soft tissue and bone cultures are imperative to reliably determine infectious organisms, whereas superficial cultures usually remain inconclusive.[30] Furthermore, bone biopsy provides definitive diagnosis for cases of osteomyelitis.

MICROBIOLOGY

Pathogenic organisms involved in pedal puncture wounds are frequently related to the specific environment in which the penetrating trauma occurred. In addition, clinical findings may also provide clues in identification of the pathogen. *Staphylococcus* and *Streptococcus* species are commonly implicated because these gram-positive bacteria usually colonize the skin; these organisms typically cause cellulitis and abscess formation.[18] Gram-negative bacteria including *Escherichia coli*, *Proteus mirabilis*, and *Klebsiella* species have been known to cause indolent infections of puncture wounds.[31] Osteomyelitis following pedal puncture wounds is most commonly caused by *Pseudomonas aeruginosa*.[11,18,31] *P aeruginosa* has been shown to be a commensal organism found in the inner sole of many types of shoe gear, therefore it should be considered a pathogen in all injuries occurring through shoes.[10] Puncture injuries occurring in bodies of water may involve *P aeruginosa*, *Aeromonas hydrophila*, *Vibrio* species, and/or *Mycobacterium marinum*.[18,32] *Eikenella corrodens* is part of the normal oropharyngeal and has been found to be the causative organism for some infections involving toothpick injuries.[13,33] Fungal and acid-fast organisms are infrequently implicated in infections of pedal puncture wounds, yet these should be considered in cases of unusual environmental exposure.

MEDICAL AND SURGICAL MANAGEMENT

Appropriate debridement and irrigation of a puncture wound in a timely fashion is the key for a successful outcome. Several classification systems have been designed to help guide treatment; however, further prospective, randomized clinical trials are needed to establish the efficacy of treatment protocols for pedal puncture wounds. Resnick and Fallat[34] provided management recommendations based on depth and severity of the wound; while Krych and Lavery[35] provided a scoring system that also incorporated the timing of treatment, radiographic findings, and footwear at the time of injury.

Tetanus immunization status must be reviewed and updated on initial presentation. As with any foot wound, the patient's vascular status should be thoroughly assessed based on medical history, physical examination, and further noninvasive vascular testing if warranted, to fully determine healing potential. Most puncture wounds presenting without radiographic involvement have been shown to heal uneventfully if addressed within 6 hours of injury.[36] Adequate wound evaluation for these cases without retained foreign bodies or signs of infection should be performed under local anesthesia in the clinical setting to provide thorough exploration, taking care to provide a regional block proximal to the site of the wound. The area should then be cleansed with an antiseptic solution such as povidone-iodine and saline. Although studies have shown toxic effects of povidone-iodine on fibroblasts within open wounds, diluted concentrations demonstrate beneficial properties in decreasing wound contamination.[37,38] Once superficial cleansing of the wound has been completed, the wound margins should be debrided to remove necrotic or irregular tissue. The wound is then packed open with a sterile Penrose drain or Nu Gauze to facilitate drainage, followed by application of dry sterile dressings. Nonweight-bearing status for the first 24 hours is encouraged to avoid discomfort. The patient is then closely followed with local wound care as needed.

For cases of retained foreign bodies and/or evidence of infection, thorough wound debridement, irrigation, and removal of the foreign body is recommended in the operating room setting.[11] Puncture wounds complicated by abscess formation and/or osteomyelitis require aggressive surgical debridement.[39] In addition, cases of delayed presentation in which the wound has closed over the object and those involving children usually require operative intervention for adequate treatment. Probing and coring of the wound can safely be performed in this setting to assess the extent of injury and locate the foreign body for total removal.[19] General anesthesia is usually most appropriate for patients requiring surgical removal of retained foreign bodies to allow complete exploration. Intraoperative fluoroscopy and/or ultrasonography can facilitate triangulation of foreign bodies deep within the tissues of the foot. Deep soft tissue and bone cultures, as well as bone biopsy, should be taken to guide postoperative therapy. Aerobic and anaerobic cultures with in vitro susceptibilities should always be taken; fungal cultures and acid-fast stains should be obtained based on the environment of injury or if bacterial cultures remain inconclusive.[11,40] Once the foreign body and all nonviable soft tissue and bone has been excised as indicated, deep irrigation with copious amounts of sterile saline can be performed using a pulsed lavage system. Studies have shown no significant clinical benefit with antibiotics or other antiseptic agents added to the irrigant.[36] As previously mentioned, the wound is packed open for appropriate care. Primary closure of complicated puncture wounds may be contraindicated because of the high risk of infection.[41] Nonweight-bearing status is imperative for proper off-loading of plantar wounds. Postoperative radiographic imaging should be performed to confirm complete removal of the foreign body as well as any infected bone as indicated. Close follow-up for monitoring of the wound is imperative for prevention of further complications.

Routine use of antibiotics in pedal puncture wounds remains controversial. Typically, antibiotics are indicated only for wounds with clinical evidence of infection; however, some investigators argue for the use of prophylactic antibiotics within 24 hours of injury.[42] At present there are no prospective, randomized trials that have examined the role of antibiotic prophylaxis following puncture wounds. For superficial puncture wounds that are not considered highly contaminated, a first-generation oral cephalosporin such as cephalexin can be used. For deeper contaminated wounds or those in diabetic (or otherwise immunocompromised) patients, broad-spectrum oral antibiotics are recommended such as amoxicillin/clavulanic acid, trimethoprim/sulfamethoxazole, or clindamycin with ciprofloxacin. Antipseudomonal coverage may be used for puncture injuries through shoe gear and any cases of suspected osteomyelitis.[9,11,41,42] In patients requiring surgical debridement, parenteral antibiotics such as cefazolin, ampicillin/sulbactam, piperacillin/tazobactam, clindamycin, ciprofloxacin, and cefipime are recommended for initial broad-spectrum coverage.[18] Final antibiotic selection should be tailored according to intraoperative culture and susceptibility results. In light of the increasing prevalence of antibiotic-resistant bacteria such as methicillin-resistant staphylococci and vancomycin-resistant enterococci, coverage of these organisms is decided based on risk factors of the patient.[43] In addition, careful consideration should be undertaken in selection of levaquin or ciprofloxacin owing to emerging fluoroquinolone resistance of certain *P aeruginosa* isolates.[44] Duration of antibiotic therapy has not been established for infected puncture wounds; instead, recommendations depend on the severity of infection and the patient's response to treatment. The use of antibiotic-loaded cement beads or blocks has also been reported for the treatment of pedal osteomyelitis to provide high levels of local antibiotic while decreasing the risk of systemic toxicity.[45] Regardless of the numerous agents, antibiotic therapy cannot substitute for sound debridement and irrigation techniques in the management of severe foot infections.[46]

SUMMARY

Although pedal puncture wounds are very common injuries and most patients experience relatively uncomplicated healing courses, patients and physicians should not underestimate the value of an aggressive, systematic approach to treatment. Complications encountered after these injuries can range from cellulitis to limb-threatening infection including osteomyelitis. Early diagnosis and appropriate medical and surgical management is paramount in achieving successful outcomes.

REFERENCES

1. Reinherz RP, Hong DT, Tisa LM, et al. Management of puncture wounds of the foot. J Foot Surg 1985;24:288.
2. Fitzgerald RH, Cowan JD. Puncture wounds of the foot. Orthop Clin North Am 1975;6:965.
3. Houston A, Roy WA, Faust RA, et al. Tetanus prophylaxis in the treatment of puncture wounds of patients in the deep South. J Trauma 1962;2:439–50.
4. Chang HC, Verhoeven W, Chay WM. Rubber foreign bodies in puncture wounds of the foot in patients wearing rubber-soled shoes. Foot Ankle Int 2001;22: 409–14.
5. Lavery LA, Harkless LB, Ashry HR, et al. Infected puncture wounds in adults with diabetes: risk factors for osteomyelitis. J Foot Ankle Surg 1994;33:561.
6. Armstrong DG, Lavery LA, Quebedeaux TL, et al. Surgical morbidity and the risk of amputation due to infected puncture wounds in diabetic versus nondiabetic adults. South Med J 1997;90:384.
7. Chisholm CD, Schlesser JF. Plantar puncture wounds: controversies and treatment recommendations. Ann Emerg Med 1989;18:1352–7.
8. Patzakis MJ, Wilkins J, Brien WW, et al. Wound site as predictor of complications following deep nail punctures of the foot. West J Med 1989;150:545–7.
9. Eidelman M, Bialik V, Miller Y, et al. Plantar puncture wounds in children: analysis of 80 hospitalized patients and late sequelae. Isr Med Assoc J 2003;5:268–71.
10. Fischer MC, Goldsmith JF, Gilligan PH. Sneakers as a source of *Pseudomonas aeruginosa* in children with osteomyelitis following puncture wounds. J Pediatr 1985;106:607–14.
11. Haverstock BD, Grossman JP. Puncture wounds of the foot. Evaluation and treatment. Clin Podiatr Med Surg 1999;16:583–96.
12. Montano JB, Steele MT, Watson WA. Foreign body retention in glass-caused wounds. Ann Emerg Med 1992;21:1360–3.

13. Imoisili MA, Bonwit AM, Bulas DI. Toothpick puncture injuries of the foot in children. Pediatr Infect Dis J 2004;23:80–2.

14. Gruber RP, Vistnes L, Pardoe R. The effect of commonly used antiseptics on wound healing. Plast Reconstr Surg 1975;55:472–6.

15. Lavery LA, Armstrong DG, Quebedeaux TL, et al. Normal laboratory values in the face of severe infections in diabetics and non-diabetics. Am J Med 1996;101:521–5.

16. Giles JT, Bathon JM. Serious infections associated with anticytokine therapies in the rheumatic diseases. J Intensive Care Med 2004;19:320–34.

17. American Diabetes Association. Peripheral arterial disease in people with diabetes. Diabetes Care 2003;26:3333–41.

18. Joseph WS. Infections following trauma. In: Joseph WS, editor. Handbook of lower extremity infections. 2nd edition. New York: Churchill Livingstone; 2003. p. 84–90.

19. Lammers RL, Magill T. Detection and management of foreign bodies in soft tissue. Emerg Med Clin North Am 1992;10:767–81.

20. Peterson JJ, Bancroft LW, Kransdorf MJ. Wooden foreign bodies: imaging appearance. Am J Roentgenol 2002;178:557–62.

21. Rockett MS, Gentile SC, Gudas CJ, et al. The use of ultrasonography for the detection of retained foreign bodies in the foot. J Foot Ankle Surg 1995;34: 478–84.

22. Shiels WE II, Babcock DS, Wilson JL, et al. Localization and guided removal of soft tissue foreign bodies with sonography. Am J Roentgenol 1990;155:1277–81.

23. Manthey DE, Storrow AB, Milbourn JM, et al. Ultrasound versus radiography in the detection of soft-tissue foreign bodies. Ann Emerg Med 1996;28:7–9.

24. Nyska M, Pomeranz S, Porat S. The advantage of computed tomography in locating a foreign body in the foot. J Trauma 1986;26:93–5.

25. Lau LS, Bin G, Jaovisidua S, et al. Cost effectiveness of magnetic resonance imaging in diagnosing *Pseudomonas aeruginosa* infection after puncture wound. J Foot Ankle Surg 1997;36:36–43.

26. Martin DR, Krishnamoorthy SK, Kalb B, et al. Decreased incidence of NSF in patients on dialysis after changing gadolinium contrast-enhanced MRI protocols. J Magn Reson Imaging 2010;31:440–6.

27. Gelfand MJ, Silberstein EB. Radionuclide imaging. Use in diagnosis of osteomyelitis in children. JAMA 1977;237:245–7.

28. Palestro CJ, Love C. Nuclear medicine and diabetic foot infections. Semin Nucl Med 2009;39:52–65.

29. Lavery LA, Walker SC, Harkless LB, et al. Infected puncture wounds in diabetic and nondiabetic adults. Diabetes Care 1995;18:1588–91.

30. Frykberg RG, Wittmayer B, Zgonis T. Surgical management of diabetic foot infections and osteomyelitis. Clin Podiatr Med Surg 2007;24:469–82.

31. Miller EH, Semian DW. Gram-negative osteomyelitis following puncture wounds of the foot. J Bone Joint Surg Am 1975;57:535–7.

32. Weber CA, Wertheimer SJ, Ognjan A. *Aeromonas hydrophila*—its implications in freshwater injuries. J Foot Ankle Surg 1995;34:442–6.

33. Robinson LG, Kourtis AP. Tale of a toothpick: *Eikenella corrodens* osteomyelitis. Infection 2000;28:332–3.

34. Resnick CD, Fallat LM. Puncture wounds: therapeutic considerations and a new classification. J Foot Surg 1990;29:147–53.

35. Krych SM, Lavery LA. Puncture wounds and foreign body reactions. Clin Podiatr Med Surg 1990;7:725–31.

36. McDevitt J, Gillespie M. Managing acute plantar puncture wounds. Emerg Nurse 2008;16:30–6.

37. Pudner R. Wound cleansing. Br J Community Nurs 1997;11:30–6.
38. Lammers RL, Fourre M, Callaham ML, et al. Effect of povidone-iodine and saline soaking on bacterial counts in acute, traumatic, contaminated wounds. Ann Emerg Med 1990;19:709–14.
39. Zgonis T, Stapleton JJ, Girard-Powell VA, et al. Surgical management of diabetic foot infections and amputations. AORN J 2008;87:935–46.
40. Wilson S, Cascio B, Neitzschman HR. Radiology case of the month. Nail puncture wound to the foot. *Mycobacterium chelonei* osteomyelitis. J La State Med Soc 1999;151:251–2.
41. Verdile VP, Freed HA, Gerard J. Puncture wounds to the foot. J Emerg Med 1989;7:193–9.
42. Pennycook A, Makower R, O'Donnell AM. Puncture wounds of the foot: can infective complications be avoided? J R Soc Med 1994;87:581–3.
43. Hayes DW Jr, Mandracchia VJ, Buddecke DE Jr, et al. Vancomycin-resistant Enterococci infected puncture wound to the foot. A case report. Clin Podiatr Med Surg 2000;17:159–64.
44. Lee YJ, Liu HY, Lin YC, et al. Fluoroquinolone resistance of *Pseudomonas aeruginosa* isolates causing nosocomial infection is correlated with levofloxacin but not ciprofloxacin use. Int J Antimicrob Agents 2010;35:261–4.
45. Stabile DE, Jacobs AM. Local antibiotic treatment of soft tissue and bone infections of the foot. J Am Podiatr Med Assoc 1990;80:345–53.
46. Schade VL, Roukis TS. The role of polymethylmethacrylate antibiotic-loaded cement in addition to debridement for the treatment of soft tissue and osseous infections of the foot and ankle. J Foot Ankle Surg 2010;49:55–62.

Morton's Neuroma

William R. Adams II, DPM[a,b],*

KEYWORDS

- Neuroma • Interdigital neuroma • Neuritis
- Nerve compression syndrome • Morton neuroma

The diagnosis and treatment of Morton's neuroma is common for the foot and ankle surgeon, and are included in the differential diagnosis of any patient who presents with forefoot pain. Specific symptoms of this disorder include complaints of shooting pain, numbness and/or tingling in the third and fourth digits, burning sensation, cramping, and a feeling of "walking on a lump" in the ball of the foot. Symptoms of pain with orgasm or defecation have also been reported.[1] Patients can also relate a decrease in symptoms with removal of shoe gear or massage of the forefoot.[2,3] The symptoms associated with a neuroma are typically of gradual onset and progressively get worse with time, but can be caused by trauma.[4,5] The term neuroma is a misnomer because it is not a neoplastic or proliferative process but a degenerative one.[6] The involved nerve histologically shows demyelination of its nerve fibers, fibrosis of the epineurium and endoneurium (**Figs. 1** and **2**), and densely packed whorls of collagen called Renaut bodies.[3]

ANATOMY

The anatomy of a Morton's neuroma is well known. The neuroma is actually a benign enlargement of the third common digital branch of the medial plantar nerve (**Fig. 3**). There is a communicating branch from the fourth common digital branch of the lateral plantar nerve prior to splitting into the plantar proper digital branches. This anatomy is countered by an anatomic study by Levitsky and colleagues,[7] which demonstrated absence of the communicating branch in 73.2% of the cadavers studied.[6] This nerve passes deep to the deep transverse metatarsal ligament. The enlargement or neuroma is usually located at the level of the third and fourth metatarsal heads but often can be found just distal to the metatarsal heads. In their anatomic study, Kim and colleagues[4] found that interdigital neuromas were located distal to the deep transverse metatarsal ligament in both the midstance and heel-off stage of ambulation. Other structures worth mentioning in the plantar third interspace include the third lumbrical tendon and muscle and the third plantar metatarsal artery and veins.

[a] Wound Care Center, Jackson Purchase Medical Center, Mayfield, KY, USA
[b] Advanced Foot and Ankle Clinic, 1029 Medical Center Circle, Suite 308, Mayfield, KY 42066, USA
* Advanced Foot and Ankle Clinic, 1029 Medical Center Circle, Suite 308, Mayfield, KY 42066.
E-mail address: wa1984@ymail.com

Clin Podiatr Med Surg 27 (2010) 535–545
doi:10.1016/j.cpm.2010.06.004
0891-8422/10/$ – see front matter © 2010 Elsevier Inc. All rights reserved.

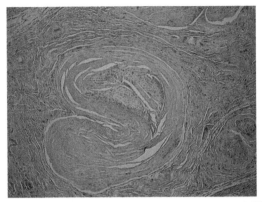

Fig. 1. Cross section of neuroma showing perineural and epineural fibrosis (hematoxylin and eosin, original magnification ×40).

HISTORY

Morton neuroma was first described by Durlacher in 1845. In 1876, Thomas G. Morton described a painful and peculiar affliction of the foot and was credited with its original description in most of the literature.[2] Morton neuroma has also been known by many names, including Morton toe, Morton metatarsalgia, Morton neuroma, interdigital neuroma, interdigital neuritis, and interdigital nerve compression syndrome.

PATHOGENESIS

Many theories have been proposed regarding the causes of this condition, which include ischemia,[8] presence of an intermetatarsal bursa,[3,9] pronation,[10] trauma,[6] and anatomic thickness of the nerve in the third interspace.[11] Recent data indicate that Morton neuroma is a nerve entrapment syndrome caused by mechanical impingement of the nerve by the deep transverse intermetatarsal ligament.[6,12,13] This observation was questioned by Kim and colleagues,[4] who found in an anatomic study that the main nerve lesion was located distal to the deep transverse metatarsal

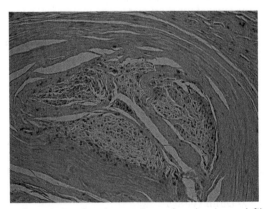

Fig. 2. Cross section of neuroma showing perineural and epineural fibrosis (hematoxylin and eosin, original magnification ×100).

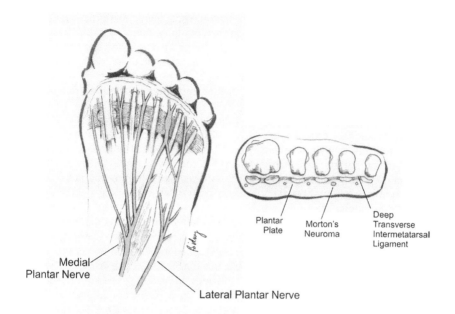

Fig. 3. Anatomy of the plantar nerves and the relationship of Morton neuroma to the deep transverse metatarsal ligament. (*From* Thomas JL, Blitch EL IV, Chaney DM, et al. Diagnosis and treatment of forefoot disorders. Section 3. Morton's intermetatarsal neuroma. J Foot Ankle Surg 2009;48(2):253; with permission.)

ligament in the both midstance and heel-off phases of gait. The investigators postulated that the condition was caused by pinching of the common digital nerve by the adjacent metatarsal heads and metatarsophalangeal joints during walking.

Barrett and Jarvis[14] pointed out that equinus deformity should be considered as a cause for nerve entrapment or neuroma. It is well established that equinus deformity increases forefoot plantar pressures. In diabetic patients, this increase in pressure is a risk factor for ulceration, which may be a contributing factor for the development of nerve entrapment or neuroma.

DIAGNOSIS

The diagnosis of Morton neuroma is mainly clinical and includes a thorough history and physical examination. The condition is more common in women than in men and is usually diagnosed between 40 and 60 years of age. A classic Mulder click can be palpated in the third interspace, with simultaneous medial to lateral compression of the forefoot with one hand and dorsal to plantar pressure on the third interspace with the opposite hand. This click is appreciated when the neuroma is pushed plantar by the third and fourth metatarsal heads.[2,3,15] A thorough examination of the metatarsophalangeal joints is helpful to rule out joint pathology. Neuroma formation can be appreciated in the second interspace but rarely in the first or fourth interspace. Most studies found the third interspace most common, but one well-documented study found an equal distribution between second and third interspace neuromas.[2]

Although the diagnosis is clinical, imaging modalities, such as radiography, magnetic resonance imaging (MRI), and ultrasonography, can play a role in diagnosis. Radiographs are mainly used to help rule out differential diagnoses such as avascular necrosis, osteoarthritis, fracture, or stress fracture. Splaying of the digits on a weight-bearing radiograph has been appreciated.[16] Some investigators believe that a neuroma can occasionally cast a faintly radiopaque shadow on plain-film radiographs.[17]

MRI can be useful to exclude other masses or pathology in the area but is not generally necessary for diagnosis of neuroma. On MRI examination, a neuroma can be seen as a mass that has low signal intensity on T1- and T2-weighted images, between or just distal to the metatarsophalangeal joints.[18] This low signal intensity results from the fibrous content of the neuroma, which distinguishes it from a neoplasm, such as a schwannoma or an intermetatarsal bursa, both of which appear hyperintense on the T2-weighted image.[19]

Ultrasonography has emerged as a valuable diagnostic tool. It is much less expensive than an MRI evaluation and can be performed in both office and hospital settings. A neuroma appears as an ovoid mass parallel to the long axis of the metatarsals. The mass has a hypoechoic signal and is best observed in the coronal view.[20–24] Ultrasound is also useful to rule out pathology of surrounding soft tissue structures quickly and easily.[25] Kankanala and Jain,[22] showed that the probability that ultrasonography will confirm the presence of plantar intermetatarsal neuroma is 91.67%. Their results revealed a sensitivity of 91.48%, a specificity of 100%, and 100% positive and 20% negative predictive values. Ultrasonography has also been used for guidance with both corticosteroid and alcohol sclerosing–type injections as treatment for intermetatarsal neuromas.[26]

Electromyography and nerve conduction velocity are useful tools when nerve pathology from a more proximal site is suspected or in patients with an atypical presentation.[3]

Other differential diagnoses that need to be excluded before treatment include tarsal tunnel syndrome, lumbar radiculopathy, peripheral neuropathy, capsulitis, bursitis, and metatarsalgia.

NONSURGICAL TREATMENT

Nonsurgical management is aimed at decreasing pressure and irritation of the nerve. This method includes avoiding high-heeled shoes and changing to a shoe with a wide toe box. Metatarsal pads placed just proximal to the metatarsal heads can help alleviate pressure and assist in spreading the metatarsal heads (**Fig. 4**). Orthotics can also be used. Bennett and colleagues[27] reported that 41% of the patients treated in their study improved with these measures alone. Oral nonsteroid and steroid medications may be used to decrease pain and inflammation. Corticosteroid and local anesthetic combination injection is commonly used. Typically, 1 to 3 injections are given. Success rates with corticosteroid injections vary greatly. Rassmussen and colleagues[28] found a success rate of 80% initially, but at 4-year follow-up only 11% of patients had lasting relief. Mann and Reynolds[2] found that corticosteroid injections neither provided lasting relief nor had predictable results. By contrast, Greenfield and colleagues[29] found that 80% of the patients who were studied indicated complete relief of pain or only slight pain at 2-year follow-up of a series of corticosteroid injections. Marcovic and colleagues[30] found that 26 of 39 patients (66%) had a positive outcome 9 months after a single ultrasound-guided cortisone injection. Saygi and colleagues[31] compared shoe gear modification along with a metatarsal pad with

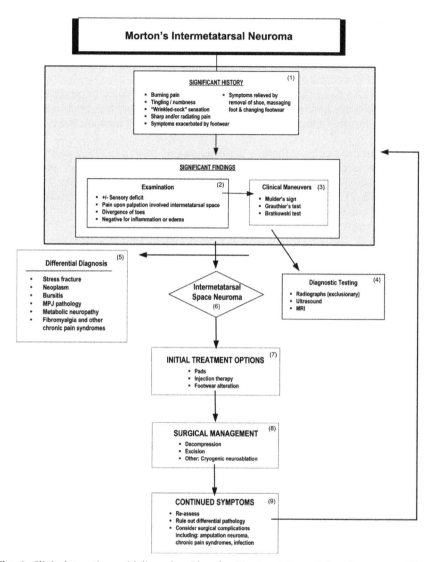

Fig. 4. Clinical practice guideline algorithm for Morton intermetatarsal neuroma. (*From* Thomas JL, Blitch EL IV, Chaney DM, et al. Diagnosis and treatment of forefoot disorders. Section 3. Morton's intermetatarsal neuroma. J Foot Ankle Surg 2009;48(2):252; with permission.)

steroid injection. These investigators found significantly higher patient satisfaction at 1, 6, and 12 months in the steroid injection group. At 12-month follow-up, 82% of those treated with steroid injections had complete or partial relief of pain compared with 63% of those with shoe gear modifications and metatarsal pads alone.

Injection of a 4% alcohol sclerosing solution has shown a success rate of 89%, with 82% of patients relaying complete relief of their symptoms. This injection was given in a series of 3 to 7 injections at 5- to 10-day intervals.[32] Several other studies have verified the effectiveness of alcohol sclerosing injections.[33,34] Corticosteroid and alcohol sclerosing injections have been used under ultrasound guidance. Hughes and colleagues[26] achieved partial or total pain relief in 94% of patients, with 84% totally pain free in a series of 101 patients undergoing alcohol sclerosing injection under ultrasound guidance. These patients had an average of 4.1 treatments and an average follow-up of 10.5 months after the last injection.

Phenol has also been described as a safe and effective injection modality for the treatment of Morton neuroma.[35] Injection of cyanocobalamin has been reported in the literature, but the effects may have been due to benzyl alcohol, the preserving agent.[36]

Extracorporeal shockwave therapy (ESWT) has also been described as an alternative to surgical excision for Morton neuroma. Fridman and colleagues[37] studied 25 patients, of whom 13 were undergoing ESWT and 12 were in a sham group. The group treated with ESWT showed a significant difference in visual analog score before and after therapy; the sham group did not have a significant difference after 12 weeks. Four of the 13 patients treated with ESWT went on to surgical excision.

SURGICAL MANAGEMENT

When conservative management fails and pain persists, surgery becomes the treatment of choice. There is debate about what type of surgery and even what approach are most effective. Surgical excision remains the most common procedure for Morton neuroma. It is most commonly performed through a dorsal or plantar longitudinal incision approach, although transverse plantar, web splitting, and Y-incision approaches have been described. There are a small number of studies that compare plantar versus dorsal approach for neurectomy. Akermark and colleagues[38] concluded that both the approaches were comparable for clinical outcome and patient satisfaction. However, there were significant differences regarding the residual sensory loss and number of complications in favor of the plantar approach. The most notable complication from the dorsal approach was 3 missed nerves.

Although these procedures are essentially the same, with the same goal of neurectomy, differences exist in the dissection as well. With the dorsal approach, all of the dorsal soft tissue structures must be mobilized (Fig. 5). The deep transverse metatarsal ligament is released (Fig. 6). A lamina spreader is typically used to spread the third and fourth metatarsals. The nerve is the identified and dissected distally to the bifurcation. The digital nerves are transected distal to the bifurcation, then followed proximally and transected as proximally as possible (Fig. 7). Amis and colleagues[39] recommended that the nerve be excised at least 3 cm proximal to the deep transverse metatarsal ligament. Postoperatively, these patients may ambulate in a surgical shoe immediately. In contrast, the dissection from a plantar approach is simple. The nerve is readily available deep to the plantar fascia, and thus traumatic dissection through the interspace and retraction of muscle and bone during the procedure is avoided. These plantar incisions should be placed in non–weight-bearing positions between the metatarsal heads. Surgeons are often tentative about making plantar incisions for fear of hypertrophic painful scars; this has not been proved in the literature. Some surgeons advocate non–weight bearing for 2 to 3 weeks after surgery. In the Akermark study, patients in the dorsal and plantar incision groups were allowed weight bearing at 2 to 3 days.[38]

Another Surgical treatment for Morton's neuroma is nerve decompression. This can be performed open, with a minimally invasive incision or endoscopically. Nerve decompression is performed by releasing the deep transverse metatarsal ligament. Proponents of this procedure point out that Morton neuroma is not a true neuroma

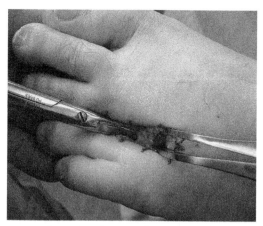

Fig. 5. Excision of neuroma by a dorsal approach. Scissor is deep into the deep transverse intermetatarsal ligament, prior to release.

but a nerve compression or entrapment syndrome. Furthermore, when the nerve is excised and resected, a true neuroma is then produced.[40–42] The endoscopic procedure described by Barrett is a 3-portal approach, with a 2.3-mm 30° scope. The dorsal portal allows for placement of a metatarsal retractor, which places tension on the deep transverse metatarsal ligament and hence allows for easier visualization and transection. A second incision is placed transversely in the web space, which allows for placement of the cannula beneath the deep transverse intermetatarsal ligament. The third incision is placed in a non–weight-bearing area of the arch through which the cannula passes as it exits the foot. Once visualized, the deep transverse intermetatarsal ligament is transected using a curved hook blade.[6,43]

In their retrospective study, Villas and colleagues[44] performed neurectomy by a dorsal approach, when macroscopic thickening of the nerve was present and observed intraoperatively. If no macroscopic changes were identified, the deep transverse intermetatarsal ligament and any other potentially compressive structure were released and the nerve was left intact. The nerve was excised in 46 of the 69 cases;

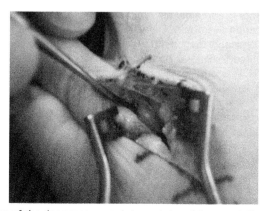

Fig. 6. After release of the deep transverse intermetatarsal ligament, the neuroma becomes easily visualized near the tip of the freer elevator.

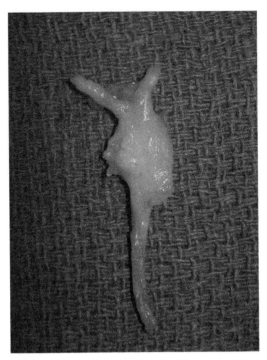

Fig. 7. Excised neuroma.

the nerve was preserved in 23 cases with release of the deep transverse metatarsal ligament. Total relief of symptoms was appreciated in all but one from each group. Both were treated successfully, with resection in the neurolysis group and more proximal resection in the neurectomy group.

Decompression with relocation has also been described.[45] With this procedure, the deep transverse intermetatarsal ligament is transected and the nerve is relocated above the ligament. A 6-0 Prolene suture is placed longitudinally through the epineurium of the nerve and tied to the periosteum or deep fascia of the adjacent metatarsal above the ligament. In this study of 82 feet in 78 patients, 95% of patients achieved complete resolution of preoperative symptoms within an average of 7 days, with full sensation restored at an average of 5 weeks.[45]

Another type of surgical management of a Morton neuroma is cryogenic neuroablation, which is a minimally invasive procedure applied at a temperature of −50°C to −70°C to the nerve. This procedure results in demyelination and ensuing wallerian degeneration of the axon, leaving the epineurium and perineurium intact. Preservation of these structures prevents the formation of stump neuromas during nerve regeneration. The drawbacks of this procedure are that the results are not permanent and that the procedure is less effective on larger neuromas or in the presence of fibrosis.[24,46]

COMPLICATIONS

Surgical treatment of Morton neuroma is not without complications. The most reported and discussed complication is recurrent or stump neuroma, which may be caused by not resecting the nerve proximal enough, incomplete excision, or tethering of the nerve to the plantar aspect of the metatarsophalangeal joint or other structures.

Typically, revisional surgery is performed through a plantar approach. Several surgeons advocate implantation of the proximal end of the nerve into an intrinsic muscle in the arch of the foot.[40,42,47] Wolfort and Dellon[47] found an additional diagnosis of tarsal tunnel syndrome in 54% of the patients who had recurrent Morton neuroma. It is not known whether these pathologies coexisted preoperatively or whether a misdiagnosis occurred.

Another complication is the resection of the digital artery during neurectomy. Su and colleagues,[48] in a review of 674 consecutive pathologic specimens, found that the digital artery was identified with the resected nerve in 39% of specimens. The investigators found no adverse effect from concomitant excision of the vessel, and hypothesized extensive collateralization of the digital vessels as an explanation for the lack of adverse outcome. There was no difference in the frequency of arterial removal between dorsal and plantar approaches to nerve excision.

Postoperative hammertoe formation has been observed. This condition is thought to be caused by inadvertent resection of the lumbrical tendon during the surgical procedure. Other complications have been reported and include, but are not limited to, hematoma, infection, complex regional pain syndrome, and hypertrophic or keloid scar formation.

SUMMARY

Morton neuroma is a common source of forefoot pain. This condition is more correctly termed as interdigital nerve compression and is not a true neuroma. Although the diagnosis is mainly clinical, imaging options are available to aid in diagnosis. Nerve conduction velocity and electromyography should be considered in complex cases or in the case of multiple neuromas to rule out more proximal nerve pathology. Many studies have shown excellent results with conservative measures.[26,31,32] When conservative measures fail and symptoms persist, surgical intervention is necessary. Surgical options include excision, decompression, and cryogenic neuroablation. All treatments have their benefits, drawbacks, and complications, and at this point, the procedure selection is the surgeon's preference.

REFERENCES

1. Locke RK. Pain in the foot during orgasm. A case report. J Am Podiatry Assoc 1983;73:271.
2. Mann RA, Reynolds JC. Interdigital neuroma: a critical clinical analysis. Foot Ankle 1983;3:238–43.
3. Rosenberg GA, Sferra JJ. Morton's neuroma: primary and recurrent and their treatment. Foot Ankle Clin 1998;3:473–84.
4. Kim JY, Choi JH, Park J, et al. An anatomical study of Morton's interdigital neuroma: the relationship between the occurring site and the deep transverse metatarsal ligament. Foot Ankle Int 2007;28(9):1007–10.
5. Larson EE, Barrett SL, Battiston B, et al. Accurate nomenclature for forefoot nerve entrapment: a historical perspective. J Am Podiatr Med Assoc 2005;95:298.
6. Barrett SL, Walsh AS. Endoscopic decompression of intermetatarsal nerve entrapment: a retrospective study. J Am Podiatr Med Assoc 2006;96(1):19–23.
7. Levitsky KA, Alman BA, Jevsevar DS, et al. Digital nerves of the foot: anatomical variations and implications regarding the pathogenesis of interdigital neuroma. Foot Ankle Int 1993;4:208.
8. Nissen KI. Plantar digital neuritis: Morton's metatarsalgia. J Bone Joint Surg 1948; 30:84–94.

9. Bossley CJ. The intermetatarsalphalangeal bursa: its significance in Morton's metatarsalgia. J Bone Joint Surg 1980;62:184–7.

10. Root ML, Orien WP, Weed JH. Normal and abnormal function of the foot. Los Angeles (CA): Clinical Biomechanics Corp; 1977.

11. Betts LO. Morton's metatarsalgia neuritis of the fourth distal nerve. Med J Aust 1940;1:514–5.

12. Graham CE, Graham DM. Morton's neuroma: a microscopic analysis of the interdigital neuroma. Foot Ankle Int 1984;5:150–3.

13. Shereff MJ, Grande DA. Electron microscopic analysis of the interdigital neuroma. Clin Orthop 1991;271:296–9.

14. Barrett SL, Jarvis J. Equinus deformity as a factor in forefoot nerve entrapment: treatment with endoscopic gastrocnemius recession. J Am Podiatr Med Assoc 2005;95(5):464–8.

15. Mulder JD. The causative mechanism in Morton's metatarsalgia. J Bone Joint Surg Br 1951;33:94–5.

16. Sullivan JD. Neuroma diagnosis by means x-ray evaluation. J Foot Ankle Surg 1967;6:45–6.

17. Wu KK. Morton's interdigital neuroma: a clinical review of its etiology, treatment, and results. J Foot Ankle Surg 1996;35:112–9.

18. Mendicino SS, Rockett MS. Morton's neuroma. Update on diagnosis and imaging. Clin Podiatr Med Surg 1997;14:303–11.

19. Timins ME. MR imaging of the foot and ankle. Foot Ankle Clin 2000;5:83–101.

20. Beggs I. Sonographic appearances of nerve tumors. J Clin Ultrasound 1999;27:363–8.

21. Pollack RA, Bellacosa RA, Dornbluth NC, et al. Sonographic analysis of Morton's neuroma. J Foot Surg 1992;31:534–7.

22. Kankanala G, Jain AS. The operational characteristics of ultrasonography for the diagnosis of plantar intermetatarsal neuroma. J Foot Ankle Surg 2007;46:213–7.

23. Redd RA, Peters VJ, Emery SF, et al. Morton neuroma: sonographic evaluation. Radiology 1989;171:415–7.

24. Thomas JL, Blitch EL IV, Chaney DM, et al. Diagnosis and treatment of forefoot disorders. Section 3. Morton's intermetatarsal neuroma. J Foot Ankle Surg 2009;48(2):251–6.

25. Kincaid BR, Barrett SL. Use of high-resolution ultrasound in evaluation of the forefoot to differentiate forefoot nerve entrapments. J Am Podiatr Med Assoc 2005; 95(5):429–32.

26. Hughes RJ, Ali K, Jones H, et al. Treatment of Morton's neuroma with alcohol injection under sonographic guidance: follow-up of 101 cases. Am J Roentgenol 2007;188(6):1535–9.

27. Bennett GL, Graham CE, Mauldin DM. Morton's interdigital neuroma: a comprehensive treatment protocol. Foot Ankle Int 1995;16:760–3.

28. Rassmussen MR, Kitaoka HB, Pantzer GL. Nonoperative treatment of plantar interdigital neuroma with single corticosteroid injection. Clin Orthop Relat Res 1996;326:188–93.

29. Greenfield J, Rea J Jr, Ilfeld FW. Morton's interdigital neuroma. indications for treatment by local injections versus surgery. Clin Orthop Relat Res 1984;185:142–4.

30. Marcovic M, Crichton K, Read JW, et al. Effectiveness of ultrasound-guided corticosteroid injection in the treatment of Morton's neuroma. Foot Ankle Int 2008; 29(5):483–7.

31. Saygi B, Yildirim Y, Saygi EK, et al. Morton neuroma: comparative results of two conservative methods. Foot Ankle Int 2005;26(7):556–9.

32. Dockery GL. The treatment of intermetatarsal neuromas with 4% alcohol sclerosing injections. J Foot Ankle Surg 1999;38(6):403–8.
33. Hyer CF, Mehl LR, Block AJ, et al. Treatment of recalcitrant intermetatarsal neuroma with 4% sclerosing alcohol injection. J Foot Ankle Surg 2005;44(4): 287–91.
34. Mozena JD, Clifford JT. Efficacy of chemical neurolysis for the treatment of interdigital nerve compression of the foot: a retrospective study. J Am Podiatr Med Assoc 2007;97(3):203–6.
35. Magnan B, Marangon A, Frigo A, et al. Local phenol injection in the treatment of interdigital neuritis of the foot (Morton's neuroma). Chir Organi Mov 2005;90: 371–7.
36. Steinberg MD. The use of vitamin B-12 in Morton's neuralgia. J Am Podiatr Med Assoc 1955;45:566–7.
37. Fridman R, Cain JD, Weil L Jr. Extracorporeal shockwave therapy for interdigital neuroma: a randomized, placebo-controlled, double blind trial. J Am Podiatr Med Assoc 2009;99(3):191–3.
38. Akermark C, Crone H, Saartok T, et al. Plantar versus dorsal incision in the treatment of primary intermetatarsal Morton's neuroma. Foot Ankle Int 2008;29(2): 136–41.
39. Amis JA, Siverhus SW, Liwnicz BH. An anatomic basis for recurrence after Morton's neuroma excision. Foot Ankle 1992;13:153–6.
40. Banks AS, Vito GR, Giorgini TL. Recurrent intermetatarsal neuroma: a followup study. J Am Podiatr Med Assoc 1996;86:299–306.
41. Zelent ME, Kane RM, Neese DJ, et al. Minimally invasive Morton's intermetatarsal neuroma decompression. Foot Ankle Int 2007;28(2):263–5.
42. Dellon AL. Treatment of Morton's neuroma as a nerve compression. J Am Podiatr Med Assoc 1992;82:399–402.
43. Barrett SL, Pignetti T. Endoscopic decompression for the intermetatarsal nerve entrapment: the EDIN technique: preliminary study with cadaveric specimens; early clinical results. J Foot Ankle Surg 1994;33:503.
44. Villas C, Florez B, Alfonso M. Neurectomy versus neurolysis for Morton's neuroma. Foot Ankle Int 2008;29(6):578–80.
45. Vito GR, Talarico LM. A modified technique for Morton's neuroma: decompression with relocation. J Foot Ankle Surg 2003;93(3):190–4.
46. Caporusso EF, Fallat LM, Savoy-Moore R. Cryogenic neuroablation for the treatment of lower extremity neuromas. J Foot Ankle Surg 2002;41(5):286–90.
47. Wolfort SF, Dellon AL. Treatment of recurrent neuroma of the interdigital nerve by implantation of the proximal nerve into muscle in the arch of the foot. J Foot Ankle Surg 2001;40(6):404–10.
48. Su E, Di Carlo E, O'Malley M, et al. The frequency of digital artery resection in Morton interdigital neurectomy. Foot Ankle Int 2006;27(10):801–3.

The Lisfranc Joint

D. Martin Chaney, DPM, MS

KEYWORDS

- Foot • Lisfranc • Fracture • Dislocation • Tarsometatarsal
- Metatarsal • Arthrodesis

The Lisfranc joint is named after Jacques Lisfranc de Saint-Martin, a French army field surgeon who originally described amputation through the joint.[1,2] The Lisfranc joint articulation connects the midfoot to the forefoot through multiple small articulations and a complex array of ligaments. Today, the term Lisfranc injury refers to a variety of injuries to the tarsometatarsal joint complex that involve closed or open fractures, obvious or subtle dislocations, and simple sprains. Lisfranc injuries have historically been associated with high-energy trauma such as motor vehicle accidents, industrial accidents, or crush injuries.[1] Lower-energy injuries do not create as much obvious deformity or pain. Lisfranc injuries have historically been overlooked because of the complex nature of the anatomy, common involvement with high-energy trauma, and concomitant injuries. Subtle injuries can seem innocuous but can cause long-term sequelae and hamper quality of life if not treated. It has been estimated that up to 20% of Lisfranc injuries are misdiagnosed or missed altogether.[2,3] Increased awareness of the Lisfranc anatomy and the potential for subtle injury has slowly increased the number of diagnosed injuries commonly found in everyday life and in sports.[1]

ANATOMY

The Lisfranc joint is known to encompass the tarsometatarsal articulations. The most significant portion of the joint is the articulation of the medial surface of the second metatarsal base and the lateral joint surface of the medial cuneiform. The Lisfranc ligament spans this space and is crucial to the stability of the entire tarsometatarsal joint. Surrounding musculotendinous structures provide indirect stabilization to assist in stability of this complex joint.

Anatomically, the tarsometatarsal articulations are divided into 3 synovial joints and columns. The first is the medial tarsometatarsal joint, which comprises the first metatarsal cuneiform articulation. The second and largest is the great tarsal joint. The great tarsal joint comprises the navicular-cuneiform articulations, the lateral cuneiform-cuboid articulation, the intercuneiform articulations, and the second and

---

Private Practice - Alamo Family Foot & Ankle Care, San Antonio, TX, USA
E-mail address: marty.chaney@gmail.com

Clin Podiatr Med Surg 27 (2010) 547–560
doi:10.1016/j.cpm.2010.06.005
0891-8422/10/$ – see front matter © 2010 Elsevier Inc. All rights reserved.

podiatric.theclinics.com

third metatarsal cuneiform articulations. The great tarsal joint also includes the Lisfranc articulation traversed by the Lisfranc ligament and intermetatarsal articulations of the second, third, and fourth metatarsal bases. The third synovial joint is the lateral tarsometatarsal joint or lateral column, which encompasses the fourth and fifth metatarsal articulations with the cuboid and the articulation between the fourth and fifth metatarsals.[4] The concept of these 3 synovial joints is important when using local anesthesia joint blocks to identify which joint surfaces are painful or degenerative.

The ligamentous construct of the tarsometatarsal articulations is also complex. The ligaments can be classified as dorsal, plantar, and interosseous.[5] The Lisfranc ligament is an interosseous ligament that traverses the articulation between the second metatarsal base and medial cuneiform. There are 2 other interosseous ligaments that are not commonly discussed. These 2 ligaments are located at the second metatarsal base-lateral cuneiform and fourth metatarsal-lateral cuneiform articulations. The first, third, fourth, and fifth tarsometatarsal joints have a single dorsal ligament crossing each joint, whereas the second metatarsal base has 3 dorsal ligamentous attachments to all 3 cuneiforms. The plantar ligament orientation can vary, but most commonly there are a total of 5 plantar ligaments. The first and second metatarsal bases have ligaments originating from the medial cuneiform. The third metatarsal base has a single ligament originating from the lateral cuneiform, but can also have a second plantar ligament from the medial cuneiform.[5] The fourth and fifth metatarsal bases each has a ligamentous attachment to the cuboid. There is no plantar ligament from the intermediate cuneiform to the plantar second metatarsal base. Dorsal versus plantar ligament strength has been a topic of controversy in the literature.[4,5] Biomechanical stress of these ligaments in a laboratory stetting revealed the Lisfranc ligament to be the strongest, followed by the plantar ligaments, with the dorsal tarsometatarsal ligaments being the weakest.[6]

Dorsal, plantar, and interosseous ligaments also tether the metatarsal bases to each other proximally, with the exception of the first and second metatarsal bases. There are no dorsal, plantar, or interosseous ligaments between the first and second metatarsal bases.

The second metatarsal cuneiform articulation is recessed proximally and is known as the keystone of the transverse arch or tarsometatarsal articulations. The depth of the recession can be variable.[7] It has been hypothesized that injured patients commonly exhibit shallow recessions compared with a control group. This lack of depth can be a source of instability and may be an anatomic predictor of injury potential.[7] Motion across these joints varies, with the second and third tarsometatarsal joints being the most stable.

The dorsalis pedis artery and the deep peroneal nerve traverse the Lisfranc joint between the first and second metatarsal bases. Injuries to this neurovascular bundle can compromise circulation and sensation. Distal circulation and neurologic status should be assessed to determine the need for acute reduction. The tibialis anterior tendon has its insertion on the medial column at the base of the first metatarsal and medial cuneiform. The tendon can be at risk for iatrogenic injury or be a source of frustration if it is interposed between medial and lateral cuneiforms during open or closed reduction.[2]

DEGENERATIVE JOINT DISEASE

Congenital foot structure plays an important role in the formation of nontraumatic degenerative joint disease in the Lisfranc joint. Arthrosis in the absence of trauma is less documented but is a common source of midfoot pain. Congenital and acquired deformities can contribute to midfoot or Lisfranc arthrosis. These deformities can occur in isolation or in conjunction. Hallux valgus with a short first ray or hypermobility often lend to first ray insufficiency and transfer peak pressures to the lesser metatarsals. The transfer of pressure from the first to the lesser rays can cause a myriad of painful conditions such as stress fractures, second metatarsal phalangeal joint instability, neuroma, plantar plate tears, digital deformities, and degenerative joint disease of the tarsometatarsal articulations. The second metatarsal cuneiform joint is the primary joint affected, but the other joints can also be subject to arthrosis.

Equinus is also a contributing factor that needs to evaluated and addressed, if appropriate, to reduce the stress transferred across the midfoot. Equinus contractures contributing to increased forefoot pressures are well documented in diabetic patients with neuropathy. Correction of the contracture of the posterior muscle group of the lower leg can be beneficial in preventing recurrence, nonunions, malunion, or deformity at surrounding joints of the midfoot and hindfoot.

Clinical evaluation of the painful tarsometatarsal articulation often shows first ray hypermobility with hallux rigidus or hallux valgus deformity and long second ray (**Fig. 1**).

Lesser tarsometatarsal joint disease is possible even in patients with a stable but short first ray. Palpation of the second metatarsal cuneiform joint commonly reveals hypertrophic bone and painful attempted range of motion, and can include a positive Tinel sign with percussion of the deep peroneal nerve. In patients with cavus foot structure, shoe pressure on the tarsometatarsal articulation is often a leading complaint.

The goals of surgical intervention often include reestablishing first ray stability and deformity correction. This intervention may include a first metatarsal cuneiform arthrodesis (Lapidus), proximal osteotomy, or first metatarsal phalangeal joint arthrodesis. Arthrodesis of the tarsometatarsal degenerative joints is performed similarly in patients with or without previous trauma, with the exception of the first ray. The increased intermetatarsal angle correction that is often necessary with the first ray should be addressed (**Fig. 2**).

TRAUMATIC INJURY
History

Clinical history of trauma in a variety of forms can result in the tarsometatarsal pain, instability, and dislocation with associated fractures. Low-energy trauma, such as a fall on a stair or from a height, can cause sprains or instability that may initially seem minor in comparison with high-energy injuries. High-energy causes commonly involve motor vehicle accidents or heavy equipment accidents, such as being crushed by a forklift. A tire from a motorized vehicle can apply a large amount of downward force. This force also has a large shear component that creates more soft tissue injury, and provides more transverse plane dislocations across the midfoot.

Mechanism of Injury

The mechanism of injury can involve direct or indirect trauma. The indirect mechanism is more common and often has an added rotational component. Indirect trauma usually involves an axial force on a plantarflexed foot, with subsequent external rotation of the forefoot.[8] Hyperplantarflexion injuries can also cause Lisfranc injuries if

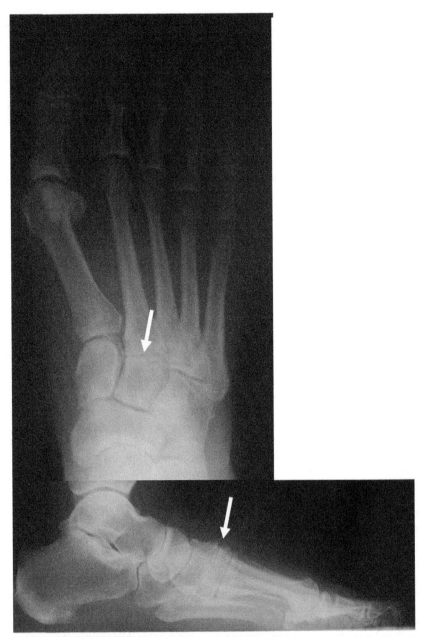

Fig. 1. Increased intermetatarsal angle, long second ray joint space narrowing, and osteophytes caused by degenerative joint disease at the second metatarsal cuneiform joint (*arrows*).

a patient's foot becomes caught under them as they fall back on the affected limb. Direct trauma involves crush injuries commonly seen in industrial accidents. I have seen the effects of a direct hit of a 7.25 kg (16-pound) bowling ball dropped on an older brother's foot, causing first and second ray dislocations.

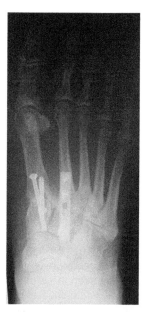

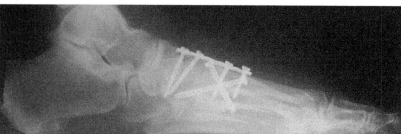

Fig. 2. Postoperative radiographs after Lapidus procedure and second metatarsal cuneiform arthrodesis.

Clinical Evaluation of the Acute and Chronic Injury

Severe injuries usually present with significant pain, obvious foot deformity, edema, and inability to bear weight. Compartment syndrome and neurovascular compromise can also be present and must be treated on an emergent basis. These types of injuries are less often missed, with the possible exception of the polytrauma patient.[8]

More subtle acute injuries can present with minimal to no obvious deformity, isolated edema, and pain with attempted ambulation. Midfoot edema and plantar ecchymosis are often present in the acute setting.[9] Low-energy injuries or injuries that have been delayed seeking treatment may present with decreased edema and no ecchymosis. There is a wide variety of presentations based on the amount of joint dislocation, joint instability, and fracture displacement. A diastasis between the hallux and second toe is possible if the first and second rays have diverged at the tarsometatarsal articulation or at the intercuneiform level. Pain with palpation can be localized to the second tarsometatarsal joint or be more generalized to the medial 3 joints. The lateral tarsometatarsal joint is less commonly involved but should also be evaluated for pain and instability. Medial or lateral stress at the metatarsal heads can be used to stress the tarsometatarsal joints and predict which joints are unstable. Myerson and colleagues[3] described the pronation abduction test, in which the forefoot is passively pronated and simultaneously abducted against a fixed hindfoot under fluoroscopy.[3]

Chronic injuries commonly have loss or decrease of the medial longitudinal arch with unstable joints that have been walked on. A single heel rise may not be possible because of instability and pain. Abduction of the forefoot with a step-off deformity at the midfoot is often visible and palpable.

Imaging

Weight-bearing anteroposterior (AP), lateral, and 30° oblique radiographs should be taken to evaluate the tarsometatarsal joint surfaces. If possible, the radiographs should be in the angle and base of gait to allow for dorsiflexion of the ankle. Non–weight-bearing radiographs can allow unstable joints to reduce. In a normal foot, the medial border of the second metatarsal base and medial border of the medial cuneiform are aligned on the AP view. The medial border of the fourth metatarsal and medial border of the cuboid should be also aligned on the oblique view. Lateral views show the superior surfaces to be aligned without a superior break in the joint line. The fleck sign is a pathognomic sign for Lisfranc injury. A small osseous fleck from the second metatarsal base or medial cuneiform can be seen representing an avulsion fracture from the Lisfranc ligament (**Fig. 3**). It can be seen in as many as 90% of cases.[2] The distance between the first and second metatarsal bases and the medial and intermediate cuneiform bones can also be helpful.[1] Contralateral views can be helpful to identify pathology when the diagnosis is uncertain or anatomic variants exist. Any diastasis greater than 2 mm of the uninjured foot can be considered diagnostic.[1]

Computed tomography (CT) and magnetic resonance imaging (MRI) are commonly used in the evaluation of Lisfranc injuries. CT is more sensitive than radiography for showing minor amounts of displacement and fractures with comminution that is often missed on plain radiographs. The strong plantar ligaments commonly cause avulsion fractures that create intra-articular fractures **Fig. 4**. These fractures are difficult to see on plain radiographs and can be a source of long-term degenerative joint pain.

MRI is especially useful to evaluate the integrity of the Lisfranc ligament. First inner-space edema or lack of visualization of the ligament can be signs of injury to the area. Rupture or partial rupture of the plantar Lisfranc ligament complex between the medial cuneiform and second and third metatarsals was shown to be a positive predictor for instability of the Lisfranc joint.[10,11] If there is a clear diastasis on weight-bearing films, MRI is not indicated. If radiographs are equivocal, then MRI can accurately disclose the degree of ligament disruption and can be a predictor for instability that may require surgery.[11]

Stress views performed under anesthesia or an ankle block can give a more accurate picture of the instability present. The foot is stabilized with one hand around the medial cuneiform and cuboid. The metatarsals are stressed with the other hand in an abduction and adduction motion under fluoroscopy to view the instability. Divergent stress to the first and second rays can also be performed to demonstrate instability. Stress views may not always be easily obtained because of the need for anesthesia, but can easily be performed after surgical intervention has already been decided on. Stress views can be helpful from a medical/legal standpoint when other imaging modalities do not adequately show the degree of instability suspected.

Classifications

Queno and Kuss[12] published their classification in 1909. Lisfranc injuries were divided into the 3 categories: homolateral, isolated, and divergent. Homolateral injuries show

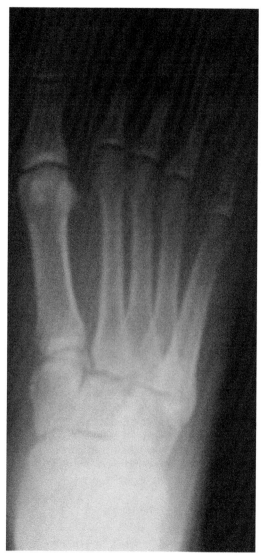

Fig. 3. Avulsion fracture from second metatarsal fleck sign indicates Lisfranc injury.

all 5 of the metatarsals dislocated in the same direction. Isolated injuries have 1 or 2 metatarsals dislocated, with the remainder remaining stable. Divergent injuries have displacement of metatarsals in different directions in sagittal and coronal planes.[2,3]

Hardcastle and colleagues[13] modified this classification in 1982 by amending the 3 categories. Homolateral or total incongruity can include medial or lateral dislocation. Isolated or partial incongruity was divided into medial and/or lateral dislocation. The divergent category shows lateral displacement of the lesser metatarsals with the first metatarsal dislocated medially. The divergent injuries can be partial or total, depending on the number of lesser metatarsals affected.

In 1986, Myerson and colleagues[3] further modified this classification system (**Fig. 5**).

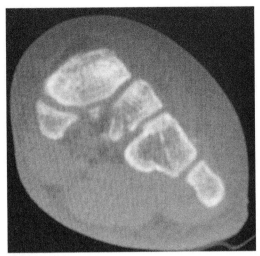

Fig. 4. Plantar intermediate cuneiform avulsion fracture from the strong plantar ligaments.

Nunley and Vertullo[14] added a classification system for Lisfranc sprains in 2002. Stage 1 shows Lisfranc ligament sprain with no diastasis of the second metatarsal base. Stage II has a ruptured Lisfranc ligament with 2- to 5-mm diastasis with no loss of arch height. Stage III shows 2- to 5-mm diastasis with loss of longitudinal arch height.

Conservative Care

In the case of a Lisfranc injury, a foot sprain is not equivalent to an ankle sprain when it comes to conservative care. Nondisplaced injuries require prolonged non–weight-bearing immobilization for at least 6 weeks. If pain continues, consider a removable boot for 4 additional weeks. This prolonged recovery time should be explained early

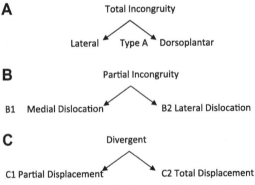

Fig. 5. (A) All the metatarsals are displaced in the same direction. (B, B1) Medial dislocation of the first ray only with lateral rays intact. (B, B2) First ray lateral dislocation and lateral dislocation of less than 4 of the lesser metatarsals. (C, C1) Medial dislocation of the first ray and lateral dislocation of less than 4 of the lesser metatarsals. (C, C2) Medial dislocation of the first ray and lateral dislocation of all 4 of the lesser metatarsals.

and often to patients who see this as a simple foot sprain that should heal much faster. Immobilization of patients with unreduced deformity generally leads to unsatisfactory outcomes and midfoot degenerative arthritis.[15] Isolated ruptures may need to be immobilized for 3 to 4 months to prevent displacement.[1] Range of motion exercises at 6 weeks can be initiated and custom orthotics are helpful as a return to normal activity is progressed. Physical therapy can be used as needed.

Decision for Surgical Intervention

The goal of surgical intervention in Lisfranc injuries should be anatomic reduction and joint stabilization. Poor anatomic reduction or lack of anatomic reduction leads to degenerative arthritis and poor patient satisfaction. The level of acceptable or unacceptable radiographic subluxation has not been definitively established. There have been many methods of measurement proposed to determine the level of subluxation. Most of these methods involve measuring the distance between the first and second metatarsal bases.[3,8,16,17] The offset distance between the medial edge of the intermediate cuneiform and the medial border of the second metatarsal also has been proposed, but much less frequently. This measurement seems intuitively more useful, but this has not been definitively proved. Open reduction with internal fixation (ORIF) has been recommended for 2 mm or more of displacement for tarsometatarsal joints, medial cuneiform second metatarsal base displacement compared with the contralateral limb.[8,18]

ORIF and Internal Fixation

Internal fixation for Lisfranc fracture dislocations has had a slow metamorphosis over many years. Kirschner-wire fixation followed by cast immobilization has been shown to be useful if anatomic reduction can be maintained throughout the immobilization process. Kirschner-wire use should be limited to primarily ligamentous injuries that can be close reduced.[15] The wires can be introduced through a percutaneous or open procedure, depending on the ease of closed reduction. Closed reduction can be aided with a bone reduction clamp providing medial force to the second metatarsal base to close the diastasis from the medial cuneiform (**Fig. 6**). Acute comminuted fractures or unstable subluxation can be stabilized with Kirschner wires, whereas less comminuted fractures can be treated with cortical or cancellous screws.[19] Dorsal plating of the medial and central columns can also be used for unstable comminuted fractures and dislocations for which wire or screw fixation is not possible. The locking and nonlocking plates available now are thinner than previous plating systems and make soft tissue coverage less precarious than it once was.

A widely used technique consists of closed or limited open reduction transarticular screw fixation across the intercuneiform articulations and first, second, and third tarsometatarsal articulations. The lateral column fourth and fifth rays can also be stabilized with transarticular screw fixation, Kirschner-wire fixation or left alone because they commonly reduce when the medial and central columns are reduced.[20] Multiple variations of internal fixation constructs have been described and are possible. An internal fixation stress study revealed that the most stable construct for the medial and central columns was a transarticular screw from the first metatarsal base to the medial cuneiform, medial cuneiform to second metatarsal base, and third metatarsal to intermediate cuneiform. According to this study, lateral column stability was not improved with screw fixation versus Kirschner-wire fixation (**Fig. 7**).[19]

Removal of internal fixation is variable, but a common recommendation is for removal of transarticular screw fixation at 6 to 12 months. This time period allows complete ligament healing and limits the chance for screw breakage or articular

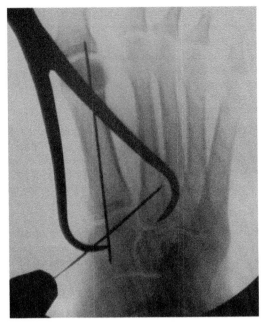

Fig. 6. Percutaneous bone clamp applied to reduce diastasis while guide wires for cannulated screws are placed.

damage to accumulate. Early screw removal at 8 weeks is prone to dislocation and recurrence of pain.

Absorbable fixation has been shown to be an acceptable form of transarticular fixation in small sample sizes for Lisfranc dislocations. The advantage is for avoidance of a secondary surgery to perform hardware removal. There were no soft tissue reactions, osteolysis, or failure of fixation in these small sample sizes.[18]

A commercial endbutton and cord system has also been reported in early studies to secure the second metatarsal base to the medial cuneiform. These systems have the advantage of not normally needing to be removed and avoiding a subsequent surgery.[17,21,22]

External fixation has also been reported to stabilize the foot in severe unstable injuries as an augment to internal fixation ORIF. Olive wire placement on the medial cuneiform and lateral fifth metatarsal bases prevents medial and lateral excursion. Lisfranc joint compression from distal to proximal can also be applied by walking the wires proximally on the foot ring when arthrodesis is desired.[20]

If open reduction is required to restore anatomic reduction of the second metatarsal base, the soft tissue or bone preventing reduction should be debrided. Ligation of the perforating branch of the dorsalis pedis may be necessary. Appropriate debridement allows reduction of the second metatarsal to oppose the medial cuneiform. Using the bone reduction clamp to hold reduction, as with percutaneous reduction, allows placement of the desired fixation.

ARTHRODESIS

The surgical approach for arthrodesis is the same as for ORIF. Percutaneous techniques during ORIF obviously limit soft tissue injury and the need for open incisions

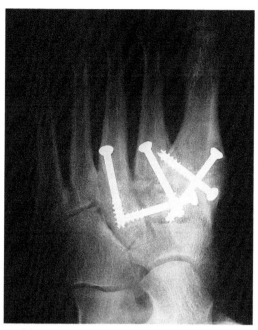

Fig. 7. Screw fixation of first, second, third metatarsal cuneiform bases, and an intercuneiform screw to stabilize intercuneiform diastasis.

if anatomic reduction can be achieved with a closed reduction. During elective surgery, I commonly approach the first metatarsal cuneiform joint from an incision dorsal and medial to the extensor hallucis long tendon. In isolation, this incision provides excellent exposure to all areas of the joint but does not allow enough exposure to reach second metatarsal cuneiform joint safely and avoid the neurovascular bundle. If a second incision is being used over the second metatarsal cuneiform joint lateral to the neurovascular bundle, I move my first ray incision more medial to ensure a sufficiently large skin bridge between the first and second ray incisions. The dorsal medial cutaneous nerve should be identified and retracted to prevent nerve damage. Full-thickness dissection allows safe protection of the neurovascular bundle between the first and second incisions.

The second ray is approached through a curved or straight incision lateral to the deep peroneal nerve and dorsalis pedis artery. The second and third metatarsal cuneiform joints can be reached through this second incision. It is common to make this incision too far medial. This error creates increased risk for deep peroneal nerve damage and may create access to the third metatarsal base. It is better to make the incision slightly more lateral than too far medial. This incision allows access to the lateral aspect of the first metarsal base through the medial fourth metatarsal base.

If needed, a third incision over the interval between the fourth and fifth metatarsal bases can be used to address the lateral column.

A transverse incision has been described to help avoid soft tissue wounds between longitudinal incisions. The incision is proximal to the arcuate artery and distal to the lateral tarsal artery. The osseous structures are approached through 6 intervals between the tendinous, nerve, and vascular structures that run perpendicular to the incision. In 12 patients, only 1 experienced wound dehiscence. This patient underwent midfoot lengthening, putting tension on the skin incision.[23]

Arthrodesis of the Lisfranc joint most commonly involves in-situ fusion of the first, second, and/or third metatarsal cuneiform joints. Increased deformity may require osteotomy, bone graft from the calcaneus or arthrodesis of navicular cuneiform joints or hindfoot joints. Adult acquired flatfoot with posterior tibial tendon dysfunction may also be present and need to be addressed with traditional procedures and those discussed earlier.

The goal in deformity reduction should include realignment of the medial border of the first metatarsal medial cuneiform, and the second metatarsal base aligned close to the medial cuneiform. The long axis of the talus and first metatarsal should also be aligned in the transverse and sagittal planes.

If possible, joint preparation should involve minimal bone resection to avoid the need for large quantities of bone graft. I typically use a combination of curved osteotomes, curettage, and, rarely, power saws. Subchondral bone should be debrided, fenestrated, or fish scaled to allow exposure to cancellous bone. Light burring with added irrigation can minimize bone loss while exposing cancellous bone. Care must be taken to avoid heat production and burning bone. Excessive bone removal can also result in metatarsal shortening and transfer metatarsalgia.

The joints can be temporarily fixated with guide pins for cannulated screw placement. Joint reduction and application should start medially and progress laterally. Temporary fixation can be applied as each joint is reduced, with final fixation applied after all joints are reduced. My preferred choice of fixation is crossing 3.5-mm or 4.0-mm screws for the first metatarsal cuneiform joint. A combination of screw and plate fixation or screw and staple fixation is also appropriate if needed as a backup. The second metatarsal can be fixated from the medial cuneiform into the second metatarsal with a cancellous or cortical screw. I recommend a second point of fixation from the second metatarsal to intermediate cuneiform screw or dorsal plate. I have used crossing screws, but the small size of the joint limits bone-to-bone contact.

Lateral Column

The fourth and fifth metatarsal cuboid articulations commonly reduce to anatomic alignment when the medial columns are reduced and fixated. It is preferable to remove scar tissue, realign the lateral column joints, and temporarily fixate with smooth wires for later removal. The lateral columns are more resistant to pain, and motion should be preserved if at all possible. Anatomic alignment is critical in the prevention of painful arthrosis and the possibility of arthrodesis. Secondary surgery where arthrodesis of the entire Lisfranc joint was fused resulted in much lower function scores that those leaving the fourth and fifth rays mobile.[24]

Arthroplasty with interposition of allograft matrix or spherical implants has been described. Long-term studies are not available and the viability of this option is not yet known, but it may be a promising alternative to arthrodesis.

ORIF Versus Primary Arthrodesis

Although the best treatment of Lisfranc fracture dislocations is not yet fully understood, I believe a general consensus exists. ORIF of a displaced Lisfranc injury pattern followed by secondary arthrodesis if pain or deformity results is the norm. This scenario seems to hold true for most trauma as it relates to the foot and ankle. As with the severely comminuted and depressed calcaneal fracture, there are likely instances for which primary arthrodesis may be the procedure of choice. The literature is slowly emerging, with studies of when to perform primary arthrodesis. ORIF has been reported to progress to osteoarthritis in from 40% to 90% of cases.[25] These patients often are converted to an arthrodesis later as a salvage procedure. Accurate anatomic alignment during ORIF is a major factor in determining which patients may in time progress to arthrosis.

Arthrodesis of the metatarsal cuneiform joints 1, 2, and 3 seems initially to do as well as ORIF in severely displaced injuries.[24,26] Patients having ORIF have higher reoperation rates when combining hardware removal and salvage arthrodesis.[25,26]

Ly and Coetzee[27] showed that patients treated with primary arthrodesis of medial 2 or 3 rays with Lisfranc ligamentous injuries excelled compared with patients having ORIF with respect to activity and pain level at 2 years.

SUMMARY

The Lisfranc joint is a complex joint encompassing 6 articulations, weak dorsal ligaments, and strong plantar ligaments. The Lisfranc ligament serves to secure the second metatarsal in the keystone of the midfoot. Traumatic ligament injury and fracture can result in deformity, instability, pain, and degenerative joint disease of the Lisfranc joint. Increased awareness of Lisfranc joint anatomy and advanced imaging has allowed more accurate diagnosis and treatment of this injured joint complex. Nontraumatic degenerative joint disease can also result from congenital and acquired deformity such as first ray insufficiency, abnormal metatarsal parabola, and equinus.

ORIF demands accurate anatomic alignment to prevent the need for salvage arthrodesis. Early studies have shown that primary arthrodesis of the medial 3 rays has performed equally well or better than ORIF for the displaced primarily ligamentous and severe injuries. A paradigm shift may emerge as more studies favor primary arthrodesis.

REFERENCES

1. DeOrio M, Erickson M, Usuelli FG, et al. Lisfranc injuries in sport. Foot Ankle Clin 2009;14(2):169–86.
2. Desmond EA, Chou LB. Current concepts review: Lisfranc injuries. Foot Ankle Int 2006;27(8):653–60.
3. Myerson MS, Fisher RT, Burgess AR, et al. Fracture dislocations of the tarsometatarsal joints: end results correlated with pathology and treatment. Foot Ankle 1986;6(5):225–42.
4. de Palma L, Santucci A, Sabetta SP, et al. Anatomy of the Lisfranc joint complex. Foot Ankle Int 1997;18(6):356–64.
5. Solan MC, Moorman CT 3rd, Miyamoto RG, et al. Ligamentous restraints of the second tarsometatarsal joint: a biomechanical evaluation. Foot Ankle Int 2001; 22(8):637–41.
6. Kura H, Luo ZP, Kitaoka HB, et al. Mechanical behavior of the Lisfranc and dorsal cuneometatarsal ligaments: in vitro biomechanical study. J Orthop Trauma 2001; 15(2):107–10.
7. Peicha G, Labovitz J, Seibert FJ, et al. The anatomy of the joint as a risk factor for Lisfranc dislocation and fracture-dislocation. An anatomical and radiological case control study. J Bone Joint Surg Br 2002;84(7):981–5.
8. Aronow MS. Treatment of the missed Lisfranc injury. Foot Ankle Clin 2006;11(1): 127–42, ix.
9. Ross G, Cronin R, Hauzenblas J, et al. Plantar ecchymosis sign: a clinical aid to diagnosis of occult Lisfranc tarsometatarsal injuries. J Orthop Trauma 1996;10(2): 119–22.

10. Raikin SM, Elias I, Dheer S, et al. Prediction of midfoot instability in the subtle Lisfranc injury. Comparison of magnetic resonance imaging with intraoperative findings. J Bone Joint Surg Am 2009;91(4):892–9.

11. Potter HG, Deland JT, Gusmer PB, et al. Magnetic resonance imaging of the Lisfranc ligament of the foot. Foot Ankle Int 1998;19(7):438–46.

12. Quenu E, Kuss G. Etude sur les luxations du metatose. Rev Chir 1909;39: 231–336.

13. Hardcastle PH, Reschauer R, Kutscha-Lissberg E, et al. Injuries to the tarsometatarsal joint. Incidence, classification and treatment. J Bone Joint Surg Br 1982; 64(3):349–56.

14. Nunley JA, Vertullo CJ. Classification, investigation, and management of midfoot sprains: Lisfranc injuries in the athlete. Am J Sports Med 2002;30(6):871–8.

15. Goossens M, De stoop N. Lisfranc's fracture-dislocations: etiology, radiology, and results of treatment. Clin Orthop Relat Res 1983;176:154–62.

16. Cassebaum WH. Lisfranc fracture-dislocations. Clin Orthop Relat Res 1963;30: 116–29.

17. Baravarian B, Geffen D. Lisfranc tightrope. Foot Ankle Spec 2009;2(5):249–50.

18. Thordarson DB, Hurvitz G. PLA screw fixation of Lisfranc injuries. Foot Ankle Int 2002;23(11):1003–7.

19. Lee CA, Birkedal JP, Dickerson EA, et al. Stabilization of Lisfranc joint injuries: a biomechanical study. Foot Ankle Int 2004;25(5):365–70.

20. Zgonis T, Roukis TS, Polyzois VD. Lisfranc fracture-dislocations: current treatment and new surgical approaches. Clin Podiatr Med Surg 2006;23(2):303–22, vi.

21. Cottom JM, Hyer CF, Berlet GC. Treatment of Lisfranc fracture dislocations with an interosseous suture button technique: a review of 3 cases. J Foot Ankle Surg 2008;47(3):250–8.

22. Lundeen G, Sara S. Technique tip: the use of a washer and suture endobutton in revision Lisfranc fixation. Foot Ankle Int 2009;30(7):713–5.

23. Vertullo CJ, Easley ME, Nunley JA. The transverse dorsal approach to the Lisfranc joint. Foot Ankle Int 2002;23(5):420–6.

24. Mulier T, Reynders P, Dereymaeker G, et al. Severe Lisfrancs injuries: primary arthrodesis or ORIF? Foot Ankle Int 2002;23(10):902–5.

25. Coetzee JC. Making sense of Lisfranc injuries. Foot Ankle Clin 2008;13(4): 695–704, ix.

26. Henning JA, Jones CB, Sietsema DL, et al. Open reduction internal fixation versus primary arthrodesis for Lisfranc injuries: a prospective randomized study. Foot Ankle Int 2009;30(10):913–22.

27. Ly TV, Coetzee JC. Treatment of primarily ligamentous Lisfranc joint injuries: primary arthrodesis compared with open reduction and internal fixation. a prospective, randomized study. J Bone Joint Surg Am 2006;88(3):514–20.

Problems, Obstacles, and Complications of Metatarsal Lengthening for the Treatment of Brachymetatarsia

Bradley M. Lamm, DPM[a],*, Monique C. Gourdine-Shaw, DPM[b,c]

KEYWORDS

- Metatarsal lengthening • Brachymetatarsia
- Distraction osteogenesis • External fixation • Short toe

Brachymetatarsia, also known as hypoplastic metatarsal, is a condition defined as premature closure of the physis yielding anatomic shortening of 1 or more metatarsals.[1–9] The causes of hypoplastic metatarsals are idiopathic, acquired, and congenital in nature, with an increased female to male predilection. Management of brachymetatarsia is challenging because the patient suffers from symptomatic biomechanical abnormalities as well as cosmetic and psychologic concerns.

Procedures used to treat brachymetatarsia, called brachymetapody when more than 1 metatarsal is involved, attempt to lengthen the metatarsal, restore the metatarsal parabola, and maintain or improve foot and digital function. A considerable number of techniques have been devised to correct brachymetatarsia: one-stage distraction with or without bone grafting, gradual distraction, lengthening the short metatarsals and shortening the long metatarsals with or without bone graft, insertion of synthetic implant, slide osteotomy with or without bone graft, and amputation of the digit.[10] Currently, distraction osteogenesis is the most accepted and the most successful treatment performed by foot and ankle surgeons for metatarsal lengthening.[11] Gradual metatarsal lengthening has been reported to improve cosmesis, shoeing, and foot and digital function by restoring the metatarsal parabola and digital

[a] International Center for Limb Lengthening, Rubin Institute for Advanced Orthopedics, Sinai Hospital of Baltimore, 2401 West Belvedere Avenue, Baltimore, MD 21215, USA
[b] United States Naval Academy, 250 Wood Road, Annapolis, MD 21402, USA
[c] Veteran Affairs Maryland Healthcare Systems, 5A119, 10 North Greene Street, Baltimore, MD 21201, USA
* Corresponding author.
E-mail address: blamm@lifebridgehealth.org

Clin Podiatr Med Surg 27 (2010) 561–582
doi:10.1016/j.cpm.2010.06.006
0891-8422/10/$ – see front matter © 2010 Elsevier Inc. All rights reserved.

podiatric.theclinics.com

position, thus decreasing associated pain. Numerous articles regarding metatarsal lengthening have been published in the last 20 years. Although one-stage procedures have been reported, most articles report gradual lengthening of the metatarsal with distraction osteogenesis.[2–9] When metatarsal lengthening of 10 mm or greater is required, gradual distraction with external fixation is recommended.[12]

Metatarsal lengthening by callus distraction offers substantial advantages.[13] Gradual metatarsal lengthening is a safe and accurate method that is predictable.[14] The patient is able to ambulate while callus distraction gradually stretches the tendons, nerves, and vessels. Bone grafting and a donor site are not needed because distraction osteogenesis allows for natural regenerate bone formation. Patients can shower or bathe and bear weight as tolerated in a surgical shoe during treatment. Gradual distraction is associated with the lowest incidence of complications.[2,15] In addition, distraction osteogenesis is the preferred technique in cases in which previous reconstructive procedures have failed. Gradual distraction with external fixation is performed in a minimally invasive fashion via a percutaneous metatarsal osteotomy, thereby maximizing the healing potential and minimizing the scarring.[9]

Studies have confirmed that external fixation restores the metatarsal length, toe position, foot and toe function, and improves cosmesis. Pain is diminished by restoring the normal metatarsal parabola and relocating and restoring toe function.[3,6,10,16–19] Even with improved methods of managing brachymetatarsia with the use of gradual metatarsal lengthening, problems, obstacles, and complications can occur.

Complications associated with the treatment of brachymetatarsia and metatarsal lengthening have been well documented and include over lengthening, nonunion, delayed union, premature consolidation, metatarsal phalangeal joint (MPJ) subluxation, MPJ stiffness, scarring, pin site infection, pseudoarthrosis, malunion, shortening, osteomyelitis, hallux abducto valgus, and toe contractures (**Table 1**).[1–11,15,16,19–28] No documented cases of digital necrosis or digital loss occurring as a complication of callus distraction were found in the literature. Two studies have attempted to classify the complications. Caton and colleagues[1] divided them into benign, serious, and severe complications, and Magnan and colleagues[2] further classified them as mechanical, biologic, and functional complications. A standardized classification of complications associated with brachymetatarsia is therefore lacking.

To our knowledge, a reproducible standardized classification of complications associated with the treatment of brachymetatarsia has not been published. In the limb-lengthening literature, Paley[29] published a standardized classification of difficulties that can arise during distraction osteogenesis. The premise of his classification is that not all adverse results during distraction osteogenesis are true complications that affect the final outcome. He further discussed that during distraction, problems and obstacles arise that are simply hurdles to completion of a successful treatment. His classification differentiates among problems, obstacles, and complications during limb lengthening with external fixation.[29] Therefore, we applied the current standardized classification for limb lengthening to metatarsal lengthening. In this article, adverse results arising during metatarsal lengthening are presented and classified. In addition, the cause of each adverse result is discussed and clinical and surgical pearls to avoid such problems, obstacles, and complications are presented.

CLASSIFICATION OF ADVERSE RESULTS

Surgical correction of brachymetatarsia has inherent risks and resultant complications. Adverse results can occur intraoperatively, perioperatively, or postoperatively. We have classified adverse results (undesirable outcomes) that occurred during

Table 1		
Adverse results can occur intraoperatively, during distraction, or postoperatively		
Intraoperative	**During Distraction**	**Postoperative**
	Pain	Pain
Direct injury to vessels/nerves	Preconsolidation	Toe/skin contracture
Incomplete osteotomy	Neurovascular compromise	Neurovascular compromise
Axial deviation	Axial deviation	Axial deviation
Subluxation at MPJ	Subluxation at MPJ	Subluxation at MPJ
Unstable external fixation	Unstable external fixation	Unstable external fixation
	Nonunion, delayed union, malunion	Nonunion, delayed union, malunion
	Edema	Edema
	Callus/regenerate bone fracture	MPJ stiffness
	Pin site infection	Hallux abductovalgus
	Broken external fixation	Pes cavus/plantarflexed metatarsal
		Osteochondritis/chondrolysis of MPJ
		Callus/regenerate bone fracture
		Scar
		Adjacent metatarsal stress fracture
		Shortening/over lengthening of metatarsal
		Dislocation
		Osteomyelitis
		Physeal arrest
		Pseudarthrosis of MPJ
		Metatarsalgia/bursitis

Abbreviation: MPJ, metatarsal phalangeal joint.

metatarsal lengthening into problems, obstacles, and complications. Adverse results that can occur during surgical management of brachymetatarsia include digital contracture, joint luxation, axial deviation, neurologic injury, vascular injury, premature and delayed consolidation, nonunion, pin site problems, loss of length of the regenerate bone, bowing, refracture, lack of toe purchase, scar, and joint stiffness.

Problems

Problems are anticipated adverse results that arise but resolve by the end of treatment without surgical intervention.

Obstacles

Obstacles are anticipated adverse results that require surgical intervention but resolve by the end of treatment.

Complications

Complications are local or systemic adverse results whereby their associated sequelae remain unresolved at the end of treatment. Not all complications interfere with the original goals of treatment. Complications are then subdivided into minor or major. Minor complications are adverse results that remain unresolved at the end of treatment but are considered to be of little significance and do not interfere with the initial goals of surgery. Major complications are adverse results that remain unresolved at the end of treatment and interfere with the original goals of treatment.

DIGITAL CONTRACTURES

Muscles generate tension during distraction, which leads to joint contractions. In cases of tibial lengthening, the triceps surae muscles, being the largest muscle group in the leg, have the greatest resistance to lengthening and can cause flexion of the knee and plantar flexion at the ankle. In comparison, the intrinsic plantar muscles of the foot can produce a plantar flexed digit during metatarsal lengthening. As the amount of metatarsal lengthening increases, the amount of muscular tension also increases, which produces a greater influence on the toe. Patients with brachymetatarsia initially present with a dorsally displaced toe and dorsal contracture of the MPJ. Therefore, controlling the MPJ position and normalizing the toe position are challenging during distraction osteogenesis of the metatarsal. If not addressed, toe contracture results.

Normal toe position involves intrinsic and extrinsic muscle balance as well as static joint restraints (ie, joint capsule, ligaments). A brachymetatarsia toe is abnormally extended at the MPJ, which creates an imbalance of the aforementioned muscles. During metatarsal lengthening, relocating and controlling the toe position is essential for a successful outcome. In previously reported metatarsal lengthening techniques, the MPJ was pinned with an axial Kirschner wire.[12,17,28] Although this technique controlled the toe position during lengthening, the MPJ became extremely stiff postoperatively. Therefore, we reduce and stabilize the toe with 2 half-pins inserted in the base of the proximal phalanx.[9] The 2 half-pins are bridged with the metatarsal external fixator to maintain toe position and distract the MPJ.[9] Toe contracture can occur if the external fixator component that attaches to the phalanx half-pin becomes loose (**Fig. 1**).

Classification of Digital Contractures

Problem—Flexion contracture of the great toe. The toe is splinted for support and physical therapy is performed during lengthening to resolve the toe contracture.
Obstacle—Flexion contracture of the great toe requiring a flexor tendon lengthening during the consolidation phase of the first metatarsal lengthening.
Complication—Residual flexion contracture of the great toe after removal of external fixation. The great toe remains stiff and flexed despite physical therapy and dynamic splinting after fixator removal.

JOINT LUXATION

It is not uncommon to acquire subluxation or dislocation of a joint during callus distraction for brachymetatarsia. Preexisting imbalanced muscles or joint incongruity predisposes the MPJ to subluxation.[3] When evaluating lateral view radiographs, increased metatarsal declination can be seen only at the distal metaphyseal-diaphyseal junction of the lesser metatarsals. The lesser metatarsal head is plantar flexed. Therefore, MPJ incongruity is present preoperatively in cases of brachymetatarsia and close monitoring during lengthening is important to avoid joint luxation. Muscle, joint capsule, and ligament imbalances also cause joint luxation during lengthening. In cases of brachymetatarsia, hyperextension of the proximal phalanx causes the interossei to sublux dorsal to the axis of the MPJ. As a result, the interossei are no longer efficient flexors of that joint thereby allowing the toe of the short metatarsal to sit dorsal.[30] During metatarsal lengthening, subluxation and dislocation of the MPJ typically occur in the

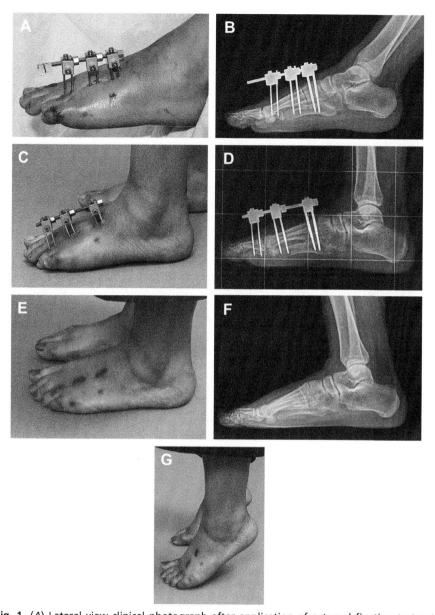

Fig. 1. (*A*) Lateral view clinical photograph after application of external fixation to treat brachymetatarsia of the fourth metatarsal. (*B*) Lateral view radiograph of brachymetatarsia of the fourth metatarsal. Note the 2 pins placed proximal and distal to the osteotomy. The pins, which determine the direction of lengthening, are placed parallel to the longitudinal axis of the fourth metatarsal. The 2 pins in the proximal phalanx distract the MPJ and maintain proper toe alignment. (*C*) Lateral view clinical photograph of the fourth digit contracted plantarly after lengthening of the fourth metatarsal for approximately 1 month after initial surgery. (*D*) Lateral view radiograph of the fourth digit contracted plantarly. The external fixator was then manually adjusted in the office to dorsiflex the toe and to reduce the contracted digit. (*E*) Lateral view clinical photograph after removal of the external fixator. (*F*) Lateral view radiograph of the fourth digit in anatomic alignment. (*G*) Lateral view clinical photograph with the patient elevated on toes shows adequate range of motion without loss of function. (Copyright 2010, Rubin Institute for Advanced Orthopedics, Sinai Hospital of Baltimore; used with permission.)

sagittal plane; however, the joint can also deviate in the transverse plane. Transverse deviation is a result of medial/lateral capsule or collateral ligament instability. More commonly, the deviation in the transverse plane occurs secondary to over lengthening of the metatarsal.

As the amount of lengthening increases or as the rate of distraction increases, so does the risk of joint luxation. Although a rapid rate of lengthening might be considered a cause of subluxation,[14] according to Masada and colleagues,[4] the most common cause of joint luxation is excessive lengthening of the metatarsal. Lengthening greater than 40% can cause serious complications.[14,31] The length of the metatarsal can also be associated with or can cause attritional rupture of the lateral collateral ligament and lateral joint capsule.[32,33] Joint luxation occurs less frequently with lengthening in younger patients because of laxity of the soft tissues.

Prophylactic pinning across the MPJ maintains digital position; however, this causes severe MPJ stiffness. In the past, the Kirschner wire was used to reposition the MPJ and maintain a rectus toe position during lengthening. When the toe was pinned plantar flexed or dorsiflexed, the digit would become stiff and would remain in this position after removal. When the toe was pinned in a dorsiflexed position after removal, the toe lacked purchase. Removing the Kirschner wire earlier did not prevent this deviation of the digit or stiffness at the MPJ.

In contrast to placing a Kirschner wire across the joint, our technique of bridging the external fixator across the MPJ allows the joint space to be maintained postoperatively.[9] The joint is then protected by distracting the MPJ by 2 to 4 mm with two 1.6-mm diameter half-pins in the proximal phalanx and bridging these half-pins to the metatarsal fixator. In addition, the toe is maintained in a rectus position during the entire lengthening.[9]

If joint subluxation occurs despite attempts to prevent it, the treatment options depend on the degree, severity, and cause. Treatment options include physiotherapy, splinting, adjustment/modification of external fixation, revision surgery, decreasing the distraction rate, and isolated capsular release of the MPJ. Untreated, unrecognized, and severe cases can entail reapplication of the external fixation or shortening of the lengthened metatarsal (**Fig. 2**).

Classification of Joint Luxation

Problem—Joint subluxation caused by rapid lengthening of the metatarsal. Decreasing the rate of distraction resolves the joint subluxation.

Obstacle—Joint subluxation requiring extension of the external fixation across the MPJ to relocate the toe and prevent recurrence of joint subluxation. The subluxation resolves before the end of treatment.

Complication—Irreducible dislocation at the MPJ after removal of the external fixation. This complication is minor if the dislocation can be resolved with physical therapy. This complication is major if residual subluxation creates pain and the foot loses function compared with the preoperative function.

AXIAL DEVIATION

Axial deviation occurs when the regenerate bone is lengthened in a deviated direction (plantar or dorsal, medial or lateral, rotated in varus or valgus). One of the causes of axial deviation of the lengthened bone is inadequate or improper placement of the external fixation construct. Typically, during the lengthening process, the fixation becomes unstable or loose, leading to plantar flexed regenerate metatarsal deviation. The deviation can be remedied by an early adjustment of the external fixation in the

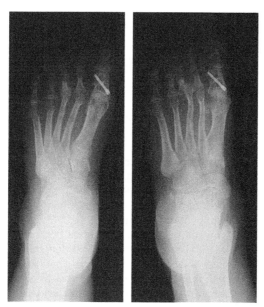

Fig. 2. Anteroposterior (*left panel*) and medial oblique (*right panel*) view radiographs of joint luxation at the third MPJ. Note that the third metatarsal was over lengthened. (Copyright 2010, Rubin Institute for Advanced Orthopedics, Sinai Hospital of Baltimore; used with permission.)

office, or by a later adjustment of the external fixation in the operating room, or by osteotomy if consolidation has occurred. On a lateral view radiograph, the dorsal cortex of the short metatarsal is parallel to the adjacent metatarsals. Improper placement of the half-pins can also lead to axial deviations. Because the external fixator is mounted perpendicular to the first or distal-most metatarsal half-pin, that pin determines the plane of lengthening. Accurately placing half-pins perpendicular to the metatarsal in the sagittal plane allows the plane of metatarsal lengthening to be such that the final position of the metatarsal head is located at the appropriate level in the sagittal plane. The second half-pin establishes the direction of metatarsal lengthening (2 fixed points determine a line) and is important because it determines the final position of the metatarsal head in the transverse plane. Placement of the second half-pin is important to ensure that the metatarsal is not lengthened into an adjacent metatarsal. To adjust the direction of lengthening, the proximal half-pin is moved slightly medial or lateral in the base of the metatarsal before insertion.

Alignment (plane and direction) during lengthening is generally unchanged, but with loss of external fixation stability, loosening of the pins, or pin drag through the skin, axial deviation of the regenerate bone can occur. Therefore, prevention or preoperative planning of axial deviation is important. Prevention of pin loosening is accomplished by simply having the patient check the device to ensure tightness. The device should always be checked in the office for any loosening. Unstable external fixation can occur with either improper technique of external fixation application or improper use of an external fixation device. The diameter, location, and insertion of half-pins determine the stability of the external fixation. For lesser metatarsal lengthening, typically 2.5-mm half-pins are used in the distal metatarsal and 3.0-mm half-pins in the proximal metatarsal. For first metatarsal lengthening, typically 3.0-mm half-pins are used to gain maximal stability. A short first metatarsal has increased declination visible on a lateral view radiograph and should be lengthened along the plane of the sole of the foot and not perpendicular to the lateral longitudinal axis as with the lesser metatarsals. Half-pins are typically placed medial on the first metatarsal, which induces medial pin drag through the skin. Pin drag causes lateral deviation of the first metatarsal during lengthening, which often is desirable to decrease the intermetatarsal angle.[5]

In addition, muscle tension can cause deviation during lengthening. In cases of tibial lengthening, the posterior and lateral leg muscles have the greatest strength and therefore greater resistance to lengthening causing procurvatum and valgus of the tibia. Similarly, the intrinsic and plantar muscles of the foot create medial and plantar flexion of the metatarsal during lengthening. With both tibial and metatarsal lengthening, the larger the amount of the lengthening, the more axial deviation occurs. Lengthening more than 40% of the metatarsal length has been reported to create a cavus deformity after distraction osteogenesis.[3]

The level of the osteotomy influences the regenerate bone and can produce axial deviation. For example, a distal tibial osteotomy with lengthening goes into varus and procurvatum. A proximal tibial osteotomy with lengthening goes into valgus and procurvatum. However, with metatarsal lengthening, the osteotomy is made at the proximal metaphyseal-diaphyseal junction or mid-diaphyseal. Both osteotomy levels can lead to similar axial deviations because the levels are so close in anatomic position. Prevention of axial deviation requires meticulous preoperative planning, adequate or proper placement of the external fixation, lengthening no more than 40% of the initial metatarsal length, and choosing the appropriate level for the osteotomy (**Figs. 3** and **4**).

Classification of Axial Deviation

Problem — Plantar or medial deviation of a metatarsal during the lengthening phase. The regenerate bone can be manipulated/repositioned during an adjustment of the external fixator in the office. The deviation resolves before the end of treatment.

Obstacle — Plantar or medial deviation treated with adjustment of the external fixator in the operating room. The deviation resolves before the end of treatment.

Complication — A healed plantar or medial deviated metatarsal lengthening that is not problematic or painful is considered a minor complication. A healed plantar or medial deviated metatarsal lengthening that causes pain and sequelae after removal is a major complication.

NEUROLOGIC INJURY

Nerve injury related to distraction is not common in repair of brachymetatarsia. However, it is wise to recognize early signs and symptoms. Neurologic insult can be associated with technique, rate of lengthening, and tension of the surrounding soft tissue on the nerve. Knowledge of the cross-sectional anatomy and layers and compartments of the foot is imperative and prevents nerve injury intraoperatively. Guidewires are inserted before half-pins for accuracy and prevention of mechanical damage to the soft tissues. In addition, neither paralytic anesthetic agents nor a tourniquet is used during the procedure to recognize a muscle contracture if the surgeon is in the proximity of a nerve.

Elicitation of paresthesias in the distribution of a nerve postoperatively may require removal of the pin. Other causes include direct injury after corticotomy, use of sagittal saw, and osteoclasis maneuver to ensure completion of the osteotomy. Compartment

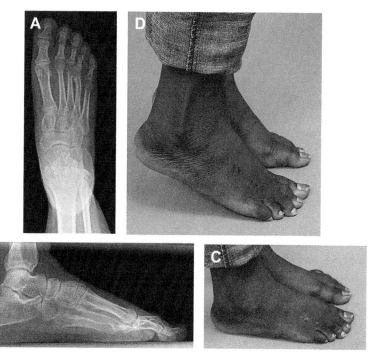

Fig. 3. (*A*) Anteroposterior view radiograph obtained after lengthening the fourth meta-tarsal. The radiograph shows medial angulation of the metatarsal. Note the metatarsal is restored to the appropriate length. (*B*) Lateral view radiograph obtained after lengthening the fourth metatarsal. The radiograph shows slight plantar angulation of the metatarsal head. (*C*) Lateral view clinical photograph. Note that there is no clinical evidence of fourth metatarsal angulation. (*D*) Lateral view clinical photograph shows no loss of function. (Copyright 2010, Rubin Institute for Advanced Orthopedics, Sinai Hospital of Baltimore; used with permission.)

syndrome, although rare in the foot without associated severe trauma, should be considered as a differential cause for nerve deficit. Symptoms of compartment syndrome progress in the following order: hyperesthesia, pain, hypoesthesia, decreased muscle strength, and paralysis. The signs and symptoms of pain and hyperesthesia should be detected and addressed early. Paralysis should not occur if the neurologic insult is treated early. If the problem results from distraction, which is rare, the rate of lengthening can be slowed or stopped. If nerve symptoms persist, prompt nerve decompression should be performed.

Classification of Neurologic Injury

Problem—Metatarsal distraction results in numbness to the toe. Decreasing the rate of distraction allows the nerve compromise to resolve before the end of treatment.
Obstacle—Metatarsal distraction results in numbness to the toe; however, decreasing the rate of distraction does not resolve the numbness. A nerve decompression is then performed, and the nerve recovers before the end of treatment.
Complication—Intraoperative nerve injuries that result in slight numbness of the toe but are not painful and do not affect the patient's shoe gear are minor complications. A major complication is a residual nerve insult that creates a neuropathic toe that remains long after treatment.

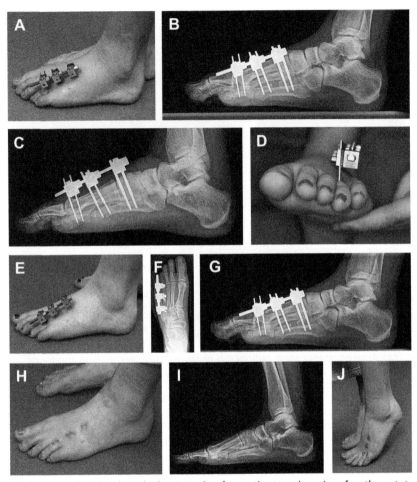

Fig. 4. (A) Lateral view clinical photograph of a patient undergoing fourth metatarsal lengthening. (B) Lateral view radiograph of the same patient undergoing fourth metatarsal lengthening. Note that the dorsal cortices are lined up and the elongated regenerate bone is in anatomic alignment. (C) Lateral view radiograph reveals the fourth metatarsal axially deviated plantarly. Note that the cortices are incongruent. (D) Anteroposterior view clinical photograph. The patient complained of a prominent plantar metatarsal head. Clinical examination revealed a prominent fourth metatarsal head and a down going fourth digit. (E) Lateral view clinical photograph after operative adjustment of the external fixator. (F) Anteroposterior view radiograph shows correction of the deformity. (G) Lateral view radiograph shows the head of the metatarsal in anatomic alignment with aligned cortices. (H) Lateral view clinical photograph after removal of external fixation. (I) Lateral view radiograph. Note the healed regenerate bone, sagittal plane alignment, and normal MPJ restoration. (J) Lateral view clinical photograph of the patient elevated on toes shows adequate range of motion. Axial deviation was corrected and therefore normal foot function was restored. No plantar prominence of fourth metatarsal head was evident on clinical examination or noted by the patient. (Copyright 2010, Rubin Institute for Advanced Orthopedics, Sinai Hospital of Baltimore; used with permission.)

VASCULAR INJURY

Vascular insult comes in many forms relative to the surgery of the distraction. Because tamponade usually corrects damage to an artery or vein, a complication that should be prevented is perforation of an artery and vein simultaneously, resulting in an arteriovenous fistula. Prevention of direct vascular insult when performing the corticotomy and limiting acute distraction at the osteotomy site decrease the incidence of hematoma. A tourniquet is not necessary during surgery because metatarsal lengthening is performed percutaneously and minimal blood loss occurs. Deep venous thrombosis can occur after any foot surgery, and patient risk factors must be elicited before surgery. Edema is a common problem as patients are allowed to bear weight as tolerated in a wooden bottom surgical shoe during the entire treatment process. The edema usually begins to resolve after the lengthening phase of treatment is completed. To prevent edema, gauze is tightly wrapped around the half-pins between the skin and external fixator. This gauze wrap is maintained at all times except showering to prevent the skin from swelling around the half-pin. If the swelling of the skin increases and decreases, the skin will move up and down the half-pin and cause irritation. This irritation can lead to a pin site infection.

Classification of Vascular Injury

Problem—Edema that is controlled with daily gauze wrapping. The daily gauze wrapping allows the edema to resolve before the end of treatment.
Obstacle—Vascular insult because of a misplaced half-pin. The half-pin should be removed and adjusted during a second surgery, which will allow the vascular insult to repair. This obstacle resolves before the end of treatment.
Complication—Nonrepairable intraoperative vascular insult that does not affect vascularity to the foot is a minor complication. Intraoperative vascular insult, deep vein thrombosis, pulmonary embolism, and compartment syndrome are major complications.

PREMATURE CONSOLIDATION

Numerous factors encourage premature consolidation, but lack of complete osteotomy is the most common cause.[29] Congenital factors favoring premature consolidation include Ollier disease and pseudohyperparathyroidism. Brachymetatarsia has been linked to several disease processes, including Down syndrome, Apert syndrome, juvenile rheumatoid arthritis, myositis ossificans, Turner syndrome, sickle cell anemia, Gorlin syndrome, hyperthyroidism, Marchesani syndrome, acrodysostosis, malignancy, Albright syndrome, and dystrophic dwarfism.[27,28,34,35] Although no correlation has been defined, the aforementioned dysplastic conditions can also cause premature consolidation.

An excessive latency period is also a causative factor of premature consolidation. One treatment option is to continue lengthening and allow the consolidated bridge to rupture. However, advise the patient that a sudden, unexpected pop with associated pain is inevitable. To prevent substantial diastasis and to decrease pain, it is necessary to reverse the distraction by the number of millimeters of distraction that have been applied since the bone consolidated. Rotational osteoclasis can be attempted in the operating room before performing repeat percutaneous corticotomy. Care must be taken to prevent the moderate bleeding that is associated with regenerate bone (**Fig. 5**).

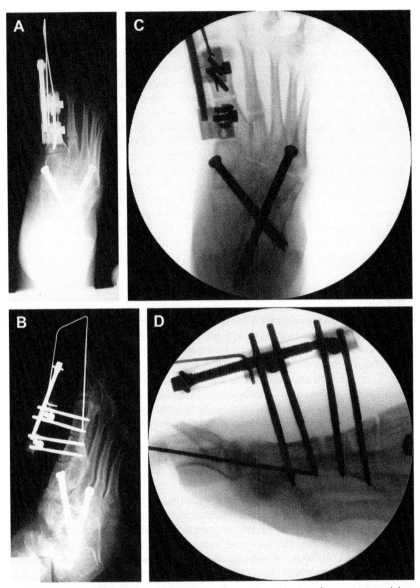

Fig. 5. (A) Anteroposterior view radiograph of a patient during first metatarsal lengthening. The radiograph does not allow for visualization of the osteotomy because of superimposition of the external fixator. This is a common occurrence on postoperative radiographs. (B) Medial oblique view radiograph. The metatarsal was lengthened for more than 14 days. Note the lack of distraction gap and the hinging on the plantar cortex. The patient reported pain at the distraction site. (C) Anteroposterior fluoroscopic view of premature consolidation of the first metatarsal. The osteotomy site was not distracted after 14 days of attempted distraction. This fluoroscopic view was obtained in the office because on the plain radiographs, the external fixator obscured the view of the osteotomy site. (D) Lateral fluoroscopic view confirmed the plantar cortex was intact, and the osteotomy was hinged by the plantar cortex (premature consolidation). A reosteotomy was performed and lengthening continued (B). (Copyright 2010, Rubin Institute for Advanced Orthopedics, Sinai Hospital of Baltimore; used with permission.)

Classification of Premature Consolidation

Problem—Nonoperative treatment of premature consolidation (ie, continue to distract).
Obstacle—Operative treatment of premature consolidation (ie, reosteotomy).
Complication—Lengthening stopped prematurely because of premature consolidation (did not obtain adequate metatarsal length) is a major complication.

DELAYED CONSOLIDATION

The causes of delayed consolidation are varied and can be separated into technical and patient factors. Technical factors include initial diastasis, instability, traumatic corticotomy, and rapid distraction. To optimize distraction and decrease the risk for delayed consolidation, damage to the periosteum and endosteum should be minimized and translation avoided at the osteotomy site. If the trabeculae are not parallel and longitudinally oriented to the distraction gap, the stability and biomechanics of the external fixation should be evaluated. Patient factors include infection, trauma, malnutrition, and metabolism. When regenerate bone healing is delayed, infection can be the primary source. Patient noncompliance can lead to traumatic insult of the regenerate bone. Patients with malnutrition or hypophosphatemic rickets (hypoparathyroidism) and those who are habitual smokers are slow to form new regenerate bone. The diagnosis of delayed regeneration is facilitated with radiographs. Ultrasonography, which is predictive for new bone formation as early as 2 weeks, is beneficial for predicting delayed consolidation.

The treatment entails reversing directions several times in an accordion fashion. This encourages the trabeculae on opposite sides of the widening interzone to become farther apart. They are then returned together and distracted at a slower rate. Sometimes, cystic changes within the regenerate bone periodically occur and are revealed by ultrasonography. If a distraction gap persists, the Wasserstein[25] or Wagner[23] method using allograph or autograph can be used to fill the distraction gap. A marked duration of time after bone grafting might be needed before removal of the external fixator. Nonoperatively, an external bone stimulator can be used along with orally administered supplemental vitamins. Dynamization or purposely weakening the stability of the external fixation over a 6-week period can encourage consolidation.

Maturation of new bone with sufficient neocorticalization must occur but might be delayed secondary to loosening of the pins in the bone. The pins can be removed if sufficient consolidation is present or exchanged intraoperatively. Stability of the external fixation is essential for regenerate bone healing.

Choice of the saw versus multiple drill osteotomy method should be considered. A saw induces increased risk of thermal necrosis of the bone. Thermal injury to the bone can cause delayed consolidation whereas a corticotomy is a low-energy osteotomy that maximizes the bone healing potential.

Some investigators have attempted to compare the rate of healing of the first metatarsal to the lesser metatarsals. The first metatarsal tends to heal faster than the lesser metatarsals[7]; however, 1 study[24] showed that the first metatarsal had a delayed healing index. We prefer lengthening lesser and first metatarsals at the same rate of 0.5 mm per day (**Fig. 6**).

Classification of Delayed Consolidation

Problem—Delayed consolidation of the metatarsal regenerate bone. This is treated with compression and redistraction. Consolidation of the metatarsal results after this nonoperative treatment.

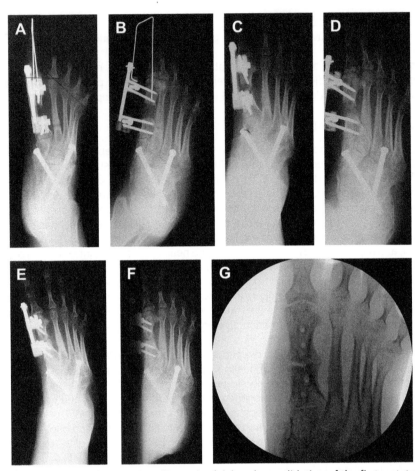

Fig. 6. (*A*) Anteroposterior view radiograph of delayed consolidation of the first metatarsal at the osteotomy. This patient was a smoker and had a scarcity of bone in the distraction gap. The rate of distraction was 0.5 mm per day. (*B*) Medial oblique view radiograph shows atrophic regenerate bone formation. (*C*) Anteroposterior view radiograph of lengthening of the first metatarsal. The regenerate bone was slowly consolidating. (*D*) Medial oblique view radiograph of the first metatarsal during lengthening. The callus has begun to consolidate. (*E*) Anteroposterior view radiograph. Three months after surgery, the regenerate bone had not consolidated. (*F*) Medial oblique view radiograph confirming incomplete consolidation of the regenerate bone. (*G*) Anteroposterior fluoroscopic view after external fixation was removed. There is evidence of delayed union along the medial cortex. (*H*) Anteroposterior view radiograph obtained after a procedure to remove the external fixator and simultaneously insert Kirschner wire fixation to strengthen the medial regenerate bone. (*I*) Medial oblique view radiograph of the first metatarsal. Note the metatarsal is out to length, and the lateral half of the metatarsal is consolidated at the distraction site. The foot was maintained in a surgical shoe for 1 month, weight bearing as tolerated, to protect the first metatarsal. (*J*) Anteroposterior view radiograph. Complete consolidation after 1 year without axial deviation. (*K*) Medial oblique view radiograph at long-term follow-up. The first metatarsal regenerate bone is completely consolidated 1 year after removal of external fixation. (Copyright 2010, Rubin Institute for Advanced Orthopedics, Sinai Hospital of Baltimore; used with permission.)

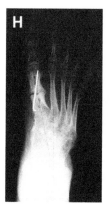
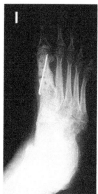
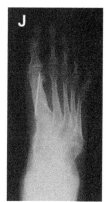
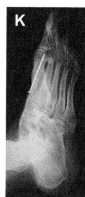

Fig. 6. (*continued*)

Obstacle—Delayed consolidation of the metatarsal. This obstacle can be managed by adding half-pins to increase the stability of the external fixation construct, allowing consolidation of the metatarsal to occur before the end of treatment.

Complication—Delayed consolidation of the metatarsal. A minor complication is treated by bone grafting, which results in a short metatarsal but does not affect the patient's goals of treatment. A major complication is treated by bone grafting and results in a short metatarsal that does affect the patient's goals of treatment.

PIN SITE PROBLEMS

Complications associated with pin site infections during distraction osteogenesis are not uncommon. Most pin site problems are attributed to associated movement of the skin relative to the pin, the amount of soft tissue between the skin and bone, and the diameter of the pin. Pin site infections, which develop from outside to inside,[29] can be minimized by maintaining adequate wire tension or pin stability. Gauze, Ilizarov sponges with antiseptic, and plain sponges act as barriers between the air and the skin. Wrapping the pins with gauze from the skin to the fixator prevents the skin from pistoning up and down the half-pin, which decreases pin site inflammation. In addition, preoperative patient education on correct pin care and external fixation adjustments is extremely important to limit pin site issues and improve the success of the lengthening.

Paley[29] developed a simple grading system for problems associated with the pin site: grade 1, soft tissue inflammation; grade 2, soft tissue infection; grade 3, bone infection. As long as grade 1 and 2 problems are addressed (usually with a 10-day course of orally administered antibiotics), serious infections associated with grade 3 do not occur. The recalcitrant infections that infect a joint/tendon or have prominent cellulitis might require pin removal with additional wire/pin placement as needed to maintain stability. Prompt action is required to prevent deep infection. Currently, small diameter half-pins are not available with hydroxyapatite coating, which would reduce the risk of loosening and thus infection (**Fig. 7**).

Classification of Pin Site Problems

Problem—Pin site infection requiring removal of the half-pin in the office and treatment with wound care and orally administered antibiotics.

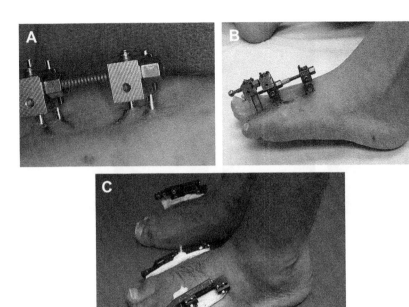

Fig. 7. (*A*) Lateral view clinical photograph of pin drag with edema. Swelling of the foot causes the pins to drag through the skin. (*B*) Lateral view clinical photograph shows superficial pin site infection around the proximal pin sites. The patient reported purulent drainage from the proximal pin sites. Note the pin drag of the 2 middle half-pins. (*C*) Lateral view clinical photograph of the gauze dressing tightly wrapped around the pin sites. The gauze prevents the skin from swelling up around the pin, which creates irritation at the pin/skin interface and causes pin site infection. In addition, the gauze prevents exposure to the outside environment and maintains cleanliness. (Copyright 2010, Rubin Institute for Advanced Orthopedics, Sinai Hospital of Baltimore; used with permission.)

Obstacle—Pin site infection requiring removal of the half-pin and addition of a new half-pin in the operating room.

Complication—Bone infection resulting from pin site infection is a major complication. Treatment of metatarsal osteomyelitis consists of bone débridement and intravenously administered antibiotics.

REFRACTURE

A major complication after removal of the external fixation construct is refracture, which commonly occurs with axial deviation of bone secondary to incomplete healing, frank fracture, and buckling of bone with loss of length. Careful evaluation of the regenerate bone before removal of the construct can prevent refracture. Neocorticalization and opacity of the regenerate bone should be similar to that of the surrounding bone. Timing for removal of the external fixator device is patient specific and varies based on multiple factors (location of osteotomy, age of patient, medical health status, medications, smoking habit, rate of lengthening, and amount of lengthening). If refracture does occur, reapplication of external fixation or casting should be considered. Refracture can also occur secondary to osteoporosis as a result of disuse, hypervascular response, or complex regional pain syndrome (**Fig. 8**).

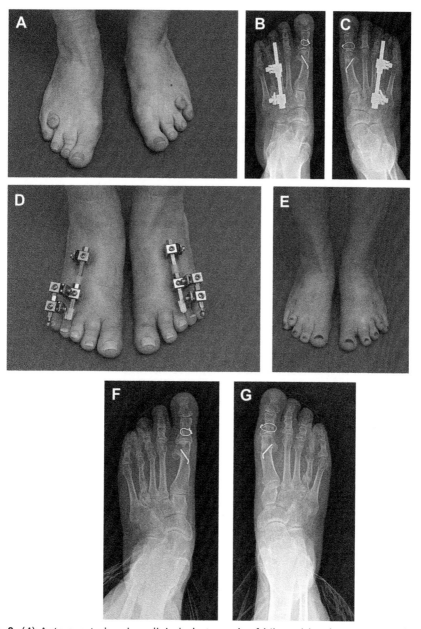

Fig. 8. (*A*) Anteroposterior view clinical photograph of bilateral brachymetatarsia of the fourth metatarsal. There is dorsal displacement of the fourth digit, and the metatarsal length is short. (*B, C*) Anteroposterior view radiograph of the left foot (*B*) and right foot (*C*) after lengthening for brachymetatarsia of the fourth metatarsal. Note the corrected metatarsal parabolas and the fourth metatarsals out to length. (*D*) Anteroposterior view clinical photograph before external fixation was removed. Note that all digits are out to length. (*E*) Anteroposterior view clinical photograph shows shortening and elevation of the fourth digits. (*F, G*) Anteroposterior view radiograph of the left foot (*F*) and right foot (*G*) after removal of the external fixator. The fourth metatarsal had shortened because of incomplete consolidation/refracture of the regenerate bone. Weight bearing was protected for 1 month after removal of the external fixator to allow for additional bone healing but resulted in a loss of metatarsal length. (Copyright 2010, Rubin Institute for Advanced Orthopedics, Sinai Hospital of Baltimore; used with permission.)

Classification of Refracture

Problem—None.
Obstacle—None.
Complication—Refracture can be a major or minor complication depending on the amount of angulation and length loss. Treatment may include reapplication of external fixation or reosteotomy for realignment.

JOINT STIFFNESS

Joint stiffness with associated loss of joint space and range of motion seems to be the most common problem associated with distraction osteogenesis for repair of brachymetatarsia.[16] Persistent muscle contractures and increased pressure on the joint during lengthening cause stiffness, which is a late complication. The effect of the temporary increased pressure on the joint is unknown. However, the functional limitation determines the severity. To prevent stiffness, the external fixation should span the joint with acute distraction. The amount of joint distraction should be 2 to 4 mm for the lesser metatarsals and 4 to 6 mm for the first MPJ. Our method of distraction osteogenesis for brachymetatarsia is combined with a spanning external fixation across the MPJ, which minimizes postoperative MPJ stiffness. We prefer to place a hinged distractor across the first MPJ to maintain joint space and motion, thus preventing the complication of joint stiffness. More importantly, motion at the MPJ is preserved when the joint is spanned, compared with Kirschner wire fixation across the joint, which creates joint scarring, cartilage damage, and does not protect the joint against joint compression when lengthening (**Fig. 9**).

Classification of Joint Stiffness

Problem—Joint stiffness managed by physical therapy, which resolves the problem before the end of treatment.
Obstacle—Joint stiffness requiring a second surgery for application of external fixation to bridge across the MPJ. The stiffness resolves before the end of treatment.
Complication—Residual MPJ stiffness after removal of the external fixation that does not affect the goal of surgery is a minor complication. Residual MPJ stiffness after removal of the external fixation that affects the patient's gait is a major complication.

OTHER PROBLEMS

Brachymetatarsia usually is not an isolated problem. Correction of associated uncompensated ankle equinus and metatarsus adductus, bunion, and nontraditional hammertoe deformity might need to be performed in cases of brachymetatarsia.

Patients who present with congenital short toes have other associated problems that need to be addressed either before or simultaneous with the lengthening. Associated problems include psychologic distress caused by the cosmetic appearance of the foot.[36] Therefore, psychologic consultations should be considered. Also, preoperative consultation regarding expectations, pain, width of the foot, residual motion, cosmesis regarding the toe and the scar, pin site care, and necessary biweekly follow-up is essential to avoid complications. The surgeon needs to be clear regarding the patient's expectations. Patients with congenital brachymetatarsia should be made aware that the toe will remain short because of shortened phalanx bones. Patients might feel that their feet are wider after metatarsal lengthening because the short metatarsal took up less forefoot shoe space. The patient should be educated regarding the potential risk of lengthening problems, obstacles, and complications.

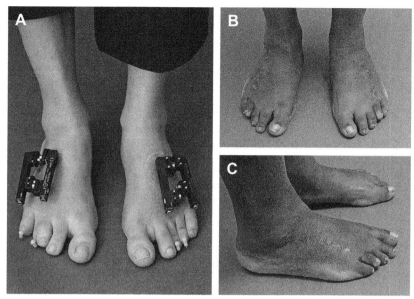

Fig. 9. (*A*) Anteroposterior view clinical photograph. Prophylactic pinning across the MPJ maintains digital position; however, this causes severe stiffness of the joint. (*B*) Anteroposterior view clinical photograph shows dorsal stiffness at the MPJ. (*C*) Lateral view clinical photograph. Note the stiffness at the MPJ, which prevents fourth digit purchase. (Copyright 2010, Rubin Institute for Advanced Orthopedics, Sinai Hospital of Baltimore; used with permission.)

Initially, the most common complaint during metatarsal lengthening is pain. The pain can be intense for the first few days or weeks. The amount of pain usually depends on multiple factors. Pain during distraction increases as the length of the regenerate bone increases. The pain can be attributed to stretching of the muscles and nerves and can be more noticeable after physical therapy, during ambulation, and in the evening. Muscle contraction from pin fixation usually resolves after a few days. If the pain interferes with sleep, oral medications for pain and sleep can be prescribed. If the pain does not resolve, decrease the rate of lengthening or prescribe oral anti-muscle spasm medications.

It is not uncommon for the patient to experience loss of appetite and/or weight. Depression, which may require a temporary course of antidepressants, usually resolves after the distraction period ends.[29] The physical and emotional pain associated with treatment should resolve after the procedure is complete, which will help the patient adjust to a normal lifestyle. Expectations and outcomes should be thoroughly discussed with patients because patient compliance and acceptance are critical to successful treatment.

DISCUSSION

We applied the current classification system for limb lengthening to distraction osteogenesis for the treatment of brachymetatarsia. Numerous adverse results are associated with metatarsal lengthening using external fixation. Adverse results are classified as problems, not complications, when they are resolved by nonoperative means.

Adverse results are classified as obstacles, not complications, when they are resolved by operative means by the end of treatment. Complications are local or systemic adverse results and their associated sequelae remain unresolved at the end of treatment. Minor complications are adverse results that remain unresolved at the end of treatment but do not interfere with the original goals of treatment. Major complications are adverse results that remain unresolved at the end of treatment and interfere with the original goals of treatment.

As opposed to the traditional brachymetatarsia treatment by stabilization of the MPJ with a Kirschner wire, our technique of acute distraction across the MPJ maintains a rectus position of the toe during lengthening and preserves function and mobility of the toe postoperatively. With the advent of our technique for bridging the MPJ, we have drastically decreased adverse results related to the MPJ and toe. In addition to the technique, the timing of the metatarsal lengthening is also important. To optimize outcomes, a patient should undergo metatarsal lengthening just after appendicular skeletal maturity (approximately age 14 years for girls and 16 years for boys).

Correction of brachymetatarsia by distraction osteogenesis can be more technically demanding than limb lengthening because of the small bones of the foot and the small external fixators that are used. A typical metatarsal lengthening is 30% to 40% of the preoperative length, which creates a challenge, just as this percentage of lengthening would for any long bone (eg, tibia, fibula, femur). Experience is required to overcome most of the problems, obstacles, and complications that are inherent to metatarsal lengthening. By presenting this classification system, we show that there are a reduced number of true complications associated with distraction osteogenesis for brachymetatarsia than previously predicted. By using this classification system, surgeons will be better prepared for surgery and for any of the aforementioned adverse results. Individualized treatment is essential, but having a clear understanding of the adverse results will offer prevention of the major complications associated with metatarsal lengthening and thus ensure successful outcomes. Postoperative MPJ function and toe mobility should not be sacrificed for additional lengthen.

REFERENCES

1. Caton J, Dumont P, Berard J, et al. Intermediate results of a series of 33 cases of leg lengthening using H. Wagner's technique. Rev Chir Orthop Reparatrice Appar Mot 1985;71(Suppl 2):44–8 [in French].
2. Magnan B, Bragantini A, Regis D, et al. Metatarsal lengthening by callotasis during the growth phase. J Bone Joint Surg Br 1995;77(4):602–7.
3. Oh CW, Satish BR, Lee ST, et al. Complications of distraction osteogenesis in short first metatarsals. J Pediatr Orthop 2004;24(6):711–5.
4. Masada K, Fujita S, Fuji T, et al. Complications following metatarsal lengthening by callus distraction for brachymetatarsia. J Pediatr Orthop 1999;19(3):394–7.
5. Lee WC, Suh JS, Moon JS, et al. Treatment of brachymetatarsia of the first and fourth ray in adults. Foot Ankle Int 2009;30(10):981–5.
6. Wilusz PM, Van P, Pupp GR. Complications associated with distraction osteogenesis for the correction of brachymetatarsia: a review of five procedures. J Am Podiatr Med Assoc 2007;97(3):189–94.
7. Erdem M, Sen C, Eralp L, et al. Lengthening of short bones by distraction osteogenesis: results and complications. Int Orthop 2009;33(3):807–13.

8. Giannini S, Faldini C, Pagkrati S, et al. One-stage metatarsal lengthening by allograft interposition: a novel approach for congenital brachymetatarsia. Clin Orthop Relat Res 2010;468(7):1933–42.
9. Lamm BM. Percutaneous distraction osteogenesis for treatment of brachymetatarsia. J Foot Ankle Surg 2010;49(2):197–204.
10. Schimizzi A, Brage M. Brachymetatarsia. Foot Ankle Clin 2004;9(3):555–70, ix.
11. Mendeszoon MJ, Kaplan YL, Crockett RS, et al. Congenital bilateral first brachymetatarsia: a case report and review of available conservative and surgical treatment options. The Foot and Ankle Online Journal 2009;2(9):1.
12. Davidson RS. Metatarsal lengthening. Foot Ankle Clin 2001;6(3):499–518.
13. Fox IM. Treatment of brachymetatarsia by the callus distraction method. J Foot Ankle Surg 1998;37(5):391–5.
14. Choi IH, Chung MS, Baek GH, et al. Metatarsal lengthening in congenital brachymetatarsia: one-stage lengthening versus lengthening by callotasis. J Pediatr Orthop 1999;19(5):660–4.
15. Gilbody J, Nayagam S. Lengthening of the first metatarsal through an arthrodesis site for treatment of brachymetatarsia: a case report. J Foot Ankle Surg 2008;47(6):559–64.
16. Lee KB, Yang HK, Chung JY, et al. How to avoid complications of distraction osteogenesis for first brachymetatarsia. Acta Orthop 2009;80(2):220–5.
17. Lamm BM. Metatarsal lengthening. In: Rozbruch RS, Ilizarov S, editors. Limb lengthening and reconstruction surgery. New York: Informa Healthcare; 2007. p. 291–302.
18. Lelievre J. Pathology of the foot. Paris: Masson; 1971 [in French].
19. Harris RI, Bearth T. The short first metatarsal: its incidence and clinical significance. J Bone Joint Surg Am 1949;31(3):553–65.
20. Lee WC, Yoo JH, Moon JS. Lengthening of fourth brachymetatarsia by three different surgical techniques. J Bone Joint Surg Br 2009;91(11):1472–7.
21. Gong HS, Jeon SH, Baek GH. Clinical tip: correction of short nail deformity in congenital brachymetatarsia by distraction lengthening. Foot Ankle Int 2009;30(5):455–7.
22. Benson JC, Banks AS. First metatarsal callus distraction. J Am Podiatr Med Assoc 2008;98(1):51–60.
23. Yamada N, Yasuda Y, Hashimoto N, et al. Use of internal callus distraction in the treatment of congenital brachymetatarsia. Br J Plast Surg 2005;58(7):1014–9.
24. Shim JS, Park SJ. Treatment of brachymetatarsia by distraction osteogenesis. J Pediatr Orthop 2006;26(2):250–4.
25. Wada A, Bensahel H, Takamura K, et al. Metatarsal lengthening by callus distraction for brachymetatarsia. J Pediatr Orthop B 2004;13(3):206–10.
26. Tomic S, Krajcinovic O, Dakic N. Use of Ilizarov mini-fixator in the treatment of congenital brachymetatarsia. Rev Chir Orthop Reparatrice Appar Mot 2000;86(2):204–8 [in French].
27. Greenfield GB. Radiology of bone diseases. 3rd edition. Philadelphia: JB Lippincott; 1982. p. 295.
28. Martin DE, Kalish SR. Brachymetatarsia: a new surgical approach. J Am Podiatr Med Assoc 1991;81(1):10–7.
29. Paley D. Problems, obstacles, and complications of limb lengthening by the Ilizarov technique. Clin Orthop Relat Res 1990;250:81–104.
30. Sarrafian SK, Topouzian LK. Anatomy and physiology of the extensor apparatus of the toes. J Bone Joint Surg Am 1969;51(4):669–79.
31. Skirving AP, Newman JH. Elongation of the first metatarsal. J Pediatr Orthop 1983;3(4):508–10.

32. Hughes J, Clark P, Klenerman L. The importance of the toes in walking. J Bone Joint Surg Br 1990;72(2):245–51.
33. Lambrinudi C. Use and abuse of toes. Postgrad Med J 1932;8(86):459–64.
34. Choudhury SN, Kitaoka HB, Peterson HA. Metatarsal lengthening: case report and review of the literature. Foot Ankle Int 1997;18(11):739–45.
35. McGlamry ED, Cooper CT. Brachymetatarsia: a surgical treatment. J Am Podiatry Assoc 1969;59(7):259–64.
36. Jimenez AL. Brachymetatarsia: a study in surgical planning. J Am Podiatry Assoc 1979;69(4):245–51.

Digital Surgery: Current Trends and Techniques

James Good, DPM*, Kyle Fiala, DPM

KEYWORDS

• Hammer toe • Claw toes • Mallet toes • Digital deformities

Hammer toes, claw toes, and mallet toes are the predominant digital deformities encountered by most foot and ankle surgeons. In recent years, increased emphasis has been placed on developing fixation for small bone and joint surgeries, especially in the foot and ankle. Specifically, the number of fixation options for the correction of digital deformities continues to expand. Although digital surgery can be rewarding for patients and surgeons alike, traditional Kirschner-wire fixation is associated with complications, often leaving the surgeon looking for better options. This article reviews the current trends in fixation of these deformities while highlighting pertinent aspects of the physical examination, radiographic examination, and surgical technique. The authors also discuss the considerations of adjunctive procedures which, when combined with these newer fixation techniques, can produce improved patient outcomes.

HISTORICAL BACKGROUND

The exact etiology of digital deformities remains multifactorial and debatable.[1] However, constrictive shoe gear has been implicated as a predominate cause.[1,2] These deformities typically develop insidiously over time and are associated with increased age. Peak incidence is generally between the fourth and the seventh decades.[1,3] Women are 4 to 5 times more likely to develop digital deformities than men.[2] Although all digits can be affected, the second toe is most commonly involved.[1–4] When appropriate conservative treatment options fail to alleviate patient complaints, surgical treatment is often warranted.

No funding was received for the support of this article.
Podiatric Medicine and Surgical Residency PM&S-36, Truman Medical Center, Lakewood, 7900 Lee's Summit Road, Kansas City, MO 64139, USA
* Corresponding author. Mid-America Foot and Ankle Specialists, P.C. Maer Building 2800 Northeast 60th Street, Gladstone, MO 64119.
E-mail address: jgood@midfoot.com

PHYSICAL EXAMINATION

A thorough physical examination is vital for a successful surgical outcome. This examination provides the basis for establishing an appropriate treatment plan. It is important to isolate the level of deformity, note which joints are involved, and identify any multiplanar deformities. Length patterns should be analyzed to ensure the most optimal functional and cosmetic outcomes. The digit should be stressed to observe for any pain, subluxation, or dislocation at the metatarsophalangeal joint (MTPJ) indicating compromised integrity of the plantar plate. Determination of the flexibility of deformity can influence procedure selection. More-advanced rigid contractures require adjunctive procedures at the metatarsal level to allow for proper correction and to maintain an intact vascular supply. Finally, the surgeon should ensure and note whether a digit purchases the ground. Many patients will be unaware of this finding preoperatively. Postoperatively, they may scrutinize the position of the digit and be unhappy with a minimally elevated but stable digital procedure.

The patient should be examined in both sitting and standing position. The flexor digitorum longus (FDL) and extensor digitorum longus (EDL) tendons should be palpated for identification of any contraction because this may need to be addressed during surgery (**Fig. 1**). The patient should be evaluated for any other contributing or corresponding deformities. Lesser digital deformities are often accompanied by hallux valgus and bunionette deformities. To achieve optimal and maintainable results, these deformities may also need to be addressed at the time of surgery.

RADIOGRAPHIC ANALYSIS

Beyond a thorough physical examination, the standard anterior-posterior, medial oblique, and lateral views are generally all that are required for analysis. Views such as forefoot axial and lateral oblique or stress radiographs may provide additional information needed for procedure selection. The classic gun-barrel sign, which is formed by the middle phalanx plantar flexing and aligning within the sagittal plane, is often pathognomonic for digital contractures. The lateral view can elucidate the degree of sagittal contracture present.

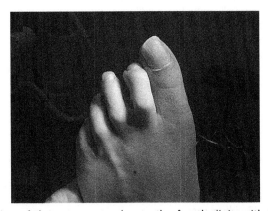

Fig. 1. Bowstringing of the extensor tendon to the fourth digit, with hammer toes and partial subluxation of the second and third MTPJs. Although clinically not symptomatic, extensor tenotomy at the MTPJ level helps to prevent any progression of this deformity postoperatively.

Attention should be focused on the overall length pattern within the foot. Excessively long or short metatarsals can be contributing factors to the development of digital deformities. The same is true for the length of the phalanges. The MTPJs should be inspected for any arthritic change, loss of joint space, subluxation, or dislocation. Most commonly, length patterns of the first and second ray should be assessed when considering first ray procedures with the correction of hammer toe deformity of the second ray (**Fig. 2**).

PROCEDURE SELECTION

The surgical management of digital deformities has historically been broken down into management of flexible or rigid deformities (**Table 1**). Practically, most digital deformities combine both fixed and flexible components presenting in a dynamic deformity. The key to achieving good outcomes involves combining the procedures to achieve the desired control at a particular joint level.

SIMPLE ARTHROPLASTY

Before surgery is discussed with the patient, it is important to have a clear understanding as to the patient's goal and expectations for the surgery. It is also important to understand the patient's current lifestyle and activity level. Although generally reserved for flexible deformities, deformities associated with skin lesions or ulcerations, and older more sedentary patients, simple arthroplasty remains a viable treatment option for addressing a myriad of digital deformities.

GENERAL SURGICAL TECHNIQUE FOR DIGITAL PROCEDURES

The patient is placed in a supine position with appropriate bolsters beneath the ipsilateral hip to address any external rotation of the extremity. A well-padded tourniquet is placed at the appropriate level, typically the ankle. Appropriate digital or ray blocks are completed without epinephrine to reduce the chance of neurovascular compromise.

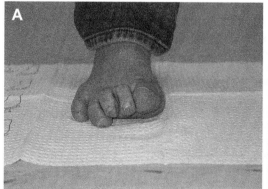 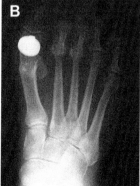

Fig. 2. (*A*) Preoperative clinical view showing significant subluxation and lack of purchase of the medial 3 digits, with a failed first MTPJ hemi-implant. (*B*) Radiograph confirming dislocation of the second and third MTPJ. Note the inherent shortening of the first metatarsal. Combined with the implant failure, this medial insufficiency produced profound lesser ray pathology.

Table 1 Procedure selection	
Flexible/Simple Deformities	**Fixed/Complex Deformities**
Flexor tenotomy	Excisional arthroplasty
Flexor-to-extensor tendon transfer	MTPJ capsulo-tendon balancing
Extensor tenotomy	Arthrodesis
Excisional arthroplasty	Distal metatarsal osteotomy (Weil osteotomy)
Derotational arthroplasty	MTPJ arthroplasty
V-Y- or Z-skin plasty	Amputation

There are numerous different incisional approaches that can be used. For digits with mild deformation, a simple transverse elliptical incision placed over the joint often works well. For more severe deformities in which an extensive soft tissue release is expected, a linear incision that extends proximal to the MTPJ provides appropriate exposure and releases the tension off the soft tissues, reducing trauma and neurovascular compromise. In patients in whom excessive shortening or tissue redundancy is to be expected, the standard, longitudinally oriented, converging, semielliptical incision remains popular among most surgeons.

Dissection of the proximal interphalangeal joint (PIPJ) is completed with the release of the medial and lateral collateral ligaments, and the head of the proximal phalanx is then resected using either hand instrumentation or a power saw for arthroplasty. When fusion is contemplated, a bone-cutting forceps is used to resect the articular surface from the head of the proximal phalanx. A rongeur can be helpful in resection of the corresponding middle phalangeal surface. An appropriate amount of bone should be removed that corresponds to the amount of deformity present. More bone resection is required for more severe deformity to limit potential neurovascular compromise. Adjacent digital length should also be taken into consideration.

The continued or altered pull of the EDL tendon can often lead to residual deformity.[5] To minimize this risk, a thorough soft tissue release should be performed proximal to the MTPJ. The EDL is stripped away from the extensor hood apparatus, leaving the periosteum intact. When capsular MTPJ release is not needed for minor deformity, stripping of the EDL can be performed subcutaneously or through a minimal incision by simply placing the scalpel blade underneath the EDL tendon parallel to the digit and gently sweeping the blade in a side-to-side motion with dorsal traction placed on the distal end of the tendon. The tendon should be released proximal to the MTPJ. If any residual deformity is still present at the MTPJ, the dorsal capsule and medial and lateral collateral ligaments should be released after the skin incision is lengthened appropriately.

If extensive MTPJ release is performed, the digit is often stabilized with Kirschner wires. In mild to moderate deformities this step may be omitted. Once all bone work has been completed, care should be taken to repair the EDL in a lengthened position. When the periosteum is left intact, this technique effectively lengthens the EDL tendon and avoids pitfalls associated with z-lengthening of a small tendon. If there is still any transverse plane deformity, the EDL tendon can also be placed on the opposite side of the deformity, further aiding transverse plane correction.

When properly indicated, performing a tenotomy of the FDL tendon can also help to decrease the risk of recurrence and add further stability. Coughlin and colleagues[1] performed flexor tenotomies for more severe cases. None of these patients went on to develop hyperextension or recurvatum, and all patients had a satisfactory outcome.

O'Kane and Kilmartin[6] reviewed the results of excisional arthroplasty performed on 100 digits for the correction of hammer toe deformities. Their study included both simple and complex fixed deformities. No release at the MTPJ level was performed, and none of the digits were stabilized with Kirschner wires. The patients were able to ambulate in normal shoe gear 2 weeks postoperatively. The results showed high levels of patient satisfaction with no major complications. A floating toe was the most common complication experienced. This excisional arthroplasty is simple, provides high patient satisfaction, and can be used to address both simple and complex deformities.

FLEXOR-TO-EXTENSOR TENDON TRANSFER

The flexor-to-extensor tendon transfer is generally indicated for flexible deformities or for added stability when other procedures are preformed.[2,5] Transferring the FDL tendon to the dorsal aspect of the proximal phalanx essentially replaces the loss of intrinsic muscular function.[2] This replacement accomplishes flexion at the MTPJ and resistance to extension at the interphalangeal joint. When used as an isolated procedure for the correction of fixed or complex deformities, the results are typically suboptimal. Complications of this procedure include toe stiffness, loss of toe flexion, floating toe, and hyperextension at the distal interphalangeal joint (DIPJ). The FDL tendon is isolated at the plantar aspect of the joint. The tendon is isolated from the split flexor digitorum brevis tendon using a hemostat. The tendon is pulled proximal and transected. The tendon is split into equal halves. Each half is clamped with a hemostat. The tendon halves are then brought around the medial and lateral sides of the proximal phalanx. Adequate tension is placed on the tendons, and the tendon halves are sutured to each other using absorbable suture. The tendon complex is then sutured into the EDL. Boyer and DeOrio[2] performed a modified version of this technique for the correction of lesser digital deformities in 79 toes. In 70 of the 79 toes (89%), the patients were satisfied with the procedure and would have it again.

SILICONE IMPLANT ARTHROPLASTY

Silicone implants for the use in foot and ankle surgery have long been the subject of debate. There are currently several different silicone implants available in the commercial market. The implants may be used as an alternative to arthroplasty or arthrodesis, as salvage for failed arthroplasty or arthrodesis, for digits that are either excessively long or short, or when space maintenance is desired. The use of the implants offers the advantage of maintaining flexibility, toe length, and shape. The placement of these implants is simpler and faster than the other procedures that are used to correct lesser digital deformities. The use of silicone implants is not without complications. Potential disadvantages include inflammatory reaction or degradation, infection, loosening of implant, loss of correction, and higher cost than traditional fixation options. Implants should be used to maintain length, and their use may be more predictable than arthroplasty. Depending on an implant to maintain alignment can lead to suboptimal outcomes.

DIGITAL ARTHRODESIS

By providing a predictable and maintainable correction, digital arthrodesis currently remains in favor among most surgeons. Numerous resection and fixation options have been described in the literature.[7] The 2 most common techniques currently used are end-to-end and peg-in-hole arthrodeses. End-to-end arthrodesis is accomplished by removing the articular surfaces of the head of the proximal phalanx and the base of the middle phalanx. The peg-in-hole technique involves inserting the head of the proximal phalanx into a peg or spike and the base of the middle phalanx into a hole or cup (**Fig. 3**). Both techniques offer distinct advantages and disadvantages. Being technically easier and faster than the peg-in-hole technique, end-to-end arthrodesis with intramedullary Kirschner-wire fixation remains the current standard among most surgeons. The use of Kirschner wires is advantageous to other forms of fixation because it offers ease of placement, simplicity, and low cost. There are, however, disadvantages to the use of Kirschner wires. Pin tract infections, breakage/bending, and lack of compression can lead to poor results and decreased patient satisfaction. With continued advancements in implant technology, newer options for fixation are available. These options offer distinct advantages over traditional fixation methods, which can further increase outcomes and patient satisfaction. Some of the newer techniques and trends are reviewed in the following sections.

CANNULATED DIGITAL FUSION SCREWS

Literature pertaining to the use of cannulated screws for interphalangeal joint arthrodesis in the foot is scarce.[3] The use of intramedullary cannulated screws for PIPJ arthrodesis for the correction of digital deformities has several advantages over other forms of fixation. External hardware is avoided, eliminating the risk of pin tract infections. Placing the screws perpendicular to the arthrodesis site maintains compression across the fusion site, potentially reducing the risk of nonunion.

The major disadvantages of the technique are screw breakage because of the relatively small diameter and long level arm, distal tuft sensitivities, a toe that is too straight, and a floating toe. Caterini and colleagues[3] used intramedullary cannulated screws for the correction of hammer toe deformities in 51 toes. At follow-up, successful arthrodesis was achieved in 48 toes (94%). The remaining toes developed a stable fibrous union. The main complications in their study were distal tuft sensitivities and screw breakage. In recent years, the authors have used cannulated screws for most of their digital arthrodesis cases and have obtained good results with minimal complications.

There are essentially 2 methods for the use of screw fixation for PIPJ arthrodesis. A small-gauge cannulated screw can be placed from the DIPJ level to stabilize the PIPJ

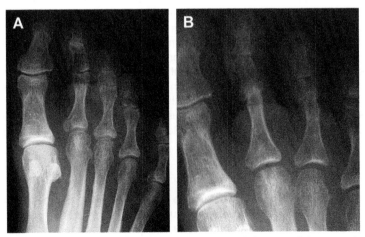

Fig. 3. (*A*) Preoperative radiograph showing hammer toe deformity of the second and third digits. (*B*) Postoperative radiograph showing stable fusions with peg-in-hole technique.

(**Fig. 4**). When successful, this method has the advantage of retained fixation and stability, avoidance of exposed wires, and more natural appearance of the digit. More commonly, fusion can be accomplished with a screw placed from the tip of the digit across both DIPJ and PIPJ (**Fig. 5**).

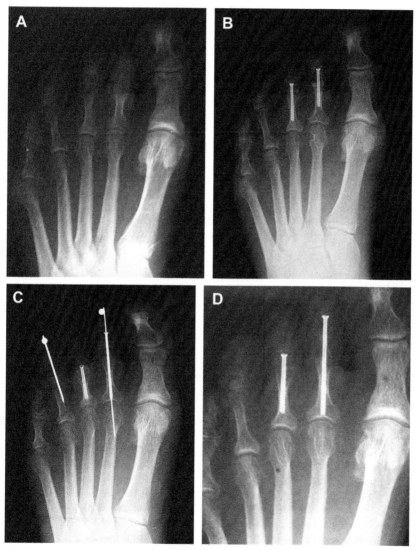

Fig. 4. (*A*) Preoperative radiograph of patient with complaints of painful second and third hammer toe deformity. (*B*) Postoperative radiograph showing DIPJ-sparing technique for second and third digital deformity. Complete consolidation across the fusion site is noted. Postoperatively, the patient developed painful mallet toe contracture of the second digit with sagittal contracture at the MTPJ, requiring additional intervention. (*C*) Early postoperative radiograph showing revision DIPJ-stabilizing technique with retained guidewire spanning the MTPJ. (*D*) Final radiograph showing stable alignment and consolidation in both digits.

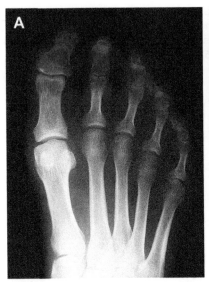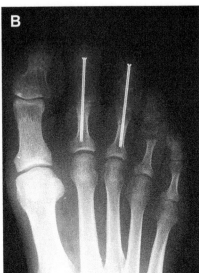

Fig. 5. (*A*) Preoperative radiograph of a patient with painful hammer toes in the second, third, and fourth digits with minimal MTPJ deformity. (*B*) Postoperative radiograph with cannulated screw fixation for second and third PIPJ arthrodesis. Resection arthroplasty was performed for the fourth-digit deformity.

DIPJ-Sparing Technique

This technique involves typical preparation of the PIPJ and release of the MTPJ as discussed previously. Attention is then directed to the DIPJ where the extensor tendon is transected and the DIPJ entered. Typically a cannulated screw is used. The guidewire is placed from the DIPJ across the fusion site.

This technique provides excellent stability and cosmetic appearance. The main postoperative complication is mallet toe contracture, which is a known complication with PIPJ arthrodesis in general. Anecdotally, using nonabsorbable braided suture for the extensor tendon repair seems to help limit this complication. Also, the guidewire can be placed across the DIPJ within the screw for a period of 2 to 4 weeks to help facilitate fibrosis and healing of the DIPJ in the corrected position.

This technique should be avoided in patients with FDL contracture unless release of this tendon is performed; if a tenotomy is not performed a mallet toe contracture may possibly ensue. Intuitively, one would expect that this technique might produce pain at the DIPJ from the screw itself. The critical portion of this technique involves adequate countersinking at the articular level of the middle phalanx. When performed appropriately, pain from the screw is rare. Mallet toe seems to be more of a problem. The senior author (James Good) has performed this approach when it was thought that patients may not tolerate screw fixation across both the PIPJ and DIPJ or when some flexion is desired at the DIPJ when severe proximal deformity might not allow complete sagittal plane correction.

DIPJ-Stabilizing Technique

The formation of a mallet toe after hammer toe repair is a troublesome and common complication, regardless of method of fixation used. Typically, the DIPJ is hyperextended when fixation is achieved with Kirschner wires in an attempt to address this issue. By placing the screw across the DIPJ, the potential for the formation of a mallet toe is avoided. At present, there are various cannulated digital fusion–specific screw sets on the market.

The standard surgical technique is used as discussed. Once the joint surfaces are prepared, temporary fixation is provided through a guidewire accompanying the screw set. The guidewire is first placed across the DIPJ in a retrograde fashion. The proximal end of the wire is then placed at the center of the medullary canal of the proximal phalanx and driven proximal to the base of the phalanx. The position of the guidewire and the arthrodesis site are checked with intraoperative fluoroscopy. A small incision is then made at the distal tip of the digit to allow passage of depth gauge and screw. The proper length of the screw is determined, which typically averages around 42 mm. The screw is then inserted from distal to proximal position across the arthrodesis site. Placement of the screw and bony apposition are confirmed fluoroscopically. Adequate compression is usually achieved without predrilling or countersinking; as a result, these steps are not routinely performed (headless screw designs will require more aggressive countersinking). The guidewire is then typically removed.

When extensive soft tissue release is performed at the MTPJ, the guidewire can be driven across the joint for added stability. The long extensor tendon is then sutured to the periosteum of the proximal phalanx in a lengthened position using absorbable suture. The incision is then closed according to the surgeon's preference, and a sterile dressing is applied. The patient is prescribed a surgical shoe and is allowed to bear weight as tolerated. A forefoot-wedge surgical shoe can be used when wire fixation crosses the MTPJ level. The patient typically uses the surgical shoe for 4 to 6 weeks or until bony consolidation is achieved. Any retained wires are usually removed at the 4-week mark.

INTRAMEDULLARY MEMORY METAL IMPLANT

The Smart Toe implant (Memometal Technologies, Bruz, France) is a one-piece metal implant designed for intramedullary fixation. The implant is composed of nitinol, a nickel-titanium alloy that expands when exposed to a higher temperature. This expansion creates compression across the arthrodesis site. The implant comes in various sizes, and can be neutral or angled with 10° of plantar flexion to give a more natural appearance to the digit (**Fig. 6**). The advantages to the use of this implant are similar to those of other forms of internal fixation. The use of these implants avoids risk of pin tract infections and pin removal, provides compression, and requires no external heat source, and the angled implant allows for a more natural appearance.

The incision, soft tissue release, and joint surface preparation are performed as previously described. Using the supplied broach, a pilot hole is made at the center of the medullary canal of the proximal phalanx. The articular cartilage is then removed from the base of the middle phalanx by the accompanying hand reamer or by any other instrument according to the surgeon's preference. Again, using the broach supplied, a pilot hole is placed at the center of the medullary canal of the middle phalanx. Next, the proper size and shape of the implant is chosen. The implant is removed from a refrigerated container and immediately placed. Using forceps to handle the implant, the proximal end is first inserted into the proximal phalanx. The distal end is then placed into the middle phalanx. Care must be taken to place the implant quickly because as the implant is warmed expansion will occur, which can lead to placement difficulties and suboptimal results. The bony surfaces are compressed until full expansion of the implant is achieved, usually for 1 to 2 minutes.

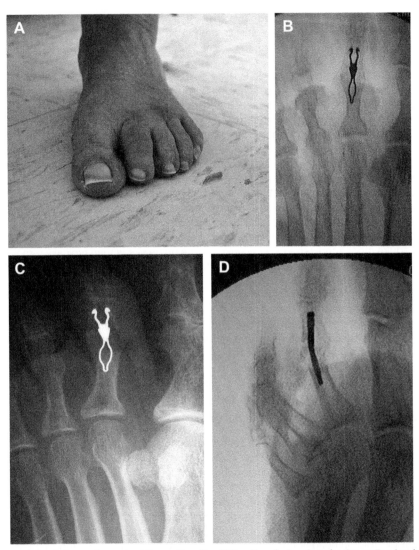

Fig. 6. (A) Left foot of a patient 3 months after PIPJ arthrodesis using the Smart Toe implant with 10° flexion. Although some swelling persists at this early juncture, the anatomic contour when compared with the adjacent digits is normal. (B) Intraoperative fluoroscopy shows the implant immediately after placement. (C) Postoperative anteroposterior radiograph showing consolidation and expansion of the implant. (D) Postoperative fluoroscopy showing the flexion within the design of the implant.

The position of the implant and apposition of arthrodesis site is confirmed fluoroscopically. The incision is then closed in the standard manner. The patient is given a surgical shoe and allowed to bear weight as tolerated for 4 to 6 weeks or until osseous union is determined.

In the authors' limited use of this implant, most results have been favorable and complications have been minor. Complications have mainly been related to improper placement of the implant. The implant must be centered within the medullary canal.

Excessive medial or lateral placement could limit compression across the arthrodesis site, cause angular deviation, or fracture the cortical wall. Aside from the normal postoperative complications, other potential complications pertaining to this implant can include malalignment, mallet toe formation, nonunion, and implant failure. Roukis[8] used this implant in 10 patients (30 toes). For 93% fusion rate, Roukis achieved successful fusion in 28 of 30 toes. The remaining toes developed a stable fibrous union. The main complications associated with the use of this implant in this study were mallet toe deformity at the DIPJ, displaced fixation, and malunion. This implant is easy, safe, and quick to use, and shows early promise.

MEMORY STAPLES

The use of staples for internal fixation has been well documented in the orthopedic literature.[9] The use of staples in foot and ankle surgery has mainly been confined to the larger joints of the foot. To the authors' knowledge, there is no literature describing the use of staples for arthrodesis of the interphalangeal joints in the toes. Traditional staples used for arthrodesis provide only static compression, which is generally insufficient for the compression needed for arthrodesis. New materials that do provide compression are now available, making this fixation option more appealing. These staples are currently offered in a smaller size, suitable for interphalangeal joint arthrodesis in the correction of lesser digital deformities. The advantages of memory staples are the avoidance of pins protruding out of the end of the toe, absence of pin tract infections, ease of placement, and dynamic compression. Disadvantages include increased cost, prominence, risk of bony injury with placement, malalignment, and the need for special equipment.

The OSStaple (BioMedical Enterprises Inc, San Antonio, TX, USA) is a staple composed of nitinol, a nickel-titanium alloy. At lower temperatures this material is pliable, and when heated the legs of the staple contract. When placed across an arthrodesis site, this contraction leads to compression (**Fig. 7**). The staple can continue to provide compression even if the bone is reabsorbed, creating dynamic compression. Dissection is performed in the usual method. Joint surfaces are

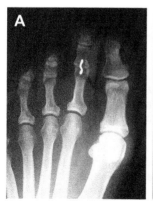 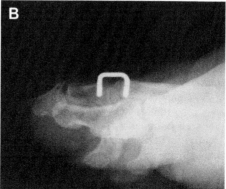

Fig. 7. (*A*) Postoperative anteroposterior radiograph showing the OSStaple implant with consolidation at the PIPJ arthrodesis site. (*B*) Lateral radiograph shows some dorsal prominence, which is a concern with this technique. Using a small burr to recess the implant can mitigate this. Any attempt at flexing the fusion site through the joint preparation leads to prominence of this fixation.

resected perpendicular to the long axis of phalanx. The appropriately sized staple is selected. The proximal hole for the staple is drilled slightly proximal to the resected joint, and the distal hole is made in a similar method. The joint surfaces are apposed, and the staple is then inserted into the corresponding drill holes using the supplied tamp. The staples are typically placed unicortically. In the past, placing the staple bicortically led to issues with painful, prominent hardware in the plantar region. The authors have found that unicortical placement provides sufficient compression across the arthrodesis site, and patients have had minimal bone healing issues with this placement. Using the supplied instrumentation, a bipolar electric current is applied to the staple. The current heats the staple, causing contraction of the legs. Visual compression of the arthrodesis site is usually observed. This technique is simple and effective, reduces soft tissue trauma, and reduces operating room time.

ABSORBABLE FIXATION

The use of absorbable fixation has successfully been used in the foot and other areas of the body.[4] Advantages to the use of these materials in lesser digital surgery for addressing digital deformities are avoidance of Kirschner wires protruding from toes, avoidance of pin tract infections, and absence of retained hardware, and they are useful for patients with metal sensitivities or allergies. Disadvantages include potential excessive swelling, lack of compression, loss of correction, mallet toe formation, and loosening of the implant. Excessive postoperative swelling and the risk of foreign body–type reactions have been concerns with the use of absorbable materials in the foot. As a result, the use of these materials has generally been low. However, newer materials have been developed, which offer promising potential. Recent research has shown that polydioxanone is degraded in the body through hydrolysis and nonspecific enzymatic activity.[4] When compared with the degradation of other forms of absorbable materials the process is slower, has fewer osteolytic changes, and has less evidence of marrow edema or inflammation.[4] These implants are typically absorbed within 24 months, which is sufficiently long enough to achieve bony consolidation. Konkel and colleagues[4] used a 2-mm absorbable pin for PIPJ arthrodesis in the correction of hammer toe deformities. The investigators achieved bony union in 38 of 48 patients (73%), and 9 of the remaining patients went on to develop a stable fibrous union. Patient satisfaction was generally high and minimal complications were encountered. Excessive swelling or foreign body–type reactions were not mentioned as a complication or source of patient dissatisfaction.

DISTAL METATARSAL OSTEOTOMY (WEIL)

The oblique capital metatarsal osteotomy, popularized by Weil, is indicated for severe long-standing digital deformity with subluxation and dislocation at the MTPJ, an excessively long metatarsal, and the need for joint decompression. This procedure is advantageous because it is stable, joint preserving, realigns the digit without undue tension on the soft tissue structures, is amenable to internal fixation, and allows for multiplanar correction (**Fig. 8**). In addition to reducing metatarsal length, the metatarsal osteotomy can be transposed medially or laterally to help balance the MTPJ (**Fig. 9**). The main disadvantages include dorsiflexion contracture at the MTPJ, transfer metatarsalgia, and reduced MTPJ range of motion. A small 3-cm incision is made directly above the joint. The EDL tendon is identified and retracted. A linear capsulotomy is made exposing the joint. The medial and lateral ligaments are released, exposing the metatarsal head. Using a sagittal saw the osteotomy is created within the dorsal one-fourth of the metatarsal head. The orientation of the osteotomy should

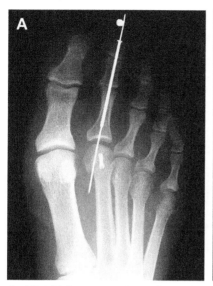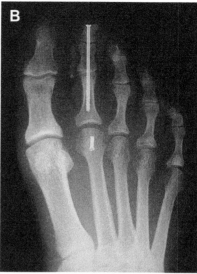

Fig. 8. (A) Initial postoperative radiograph showing cannulated screw fixation of the PIPJ arthrodesis combined with Weil osteotomy. Note the normalized metatarsal parabola. The guidewire is maintained across the MTPJ for a period of 4 weeks. (B) Final radiograph showing rectus alignment with retained screw fixation.

be as parallel to the weight-bearing surface as possible. Once the osteotomy is completed, visual proximal retraction of the metatarsal head is observed. The predetermined amount of shortening and/or angulation is applied. The osteotomy is held in place with temporary fixation. The overhang of bone created with proximal translation of the metatarsal head is excised with a rongeur. Once the position and alignment are confirmed with fluoroscopy, final fixation may be obtained. Typically this fixation is done with Kirschner wires, small-diameter screws, or absorbable materials. O'Kane and Kilmartin[10] reviewed 17 patients (20 feet) who underwent Weil osteotomy for central metatarsalgia. Fourteen of the patients (85%) were completely satisfied with the results. The main complications encountered were floating digits in 20% of the patients, and stiff or reduced motion of the MTPJ. When used as either a primary or adjunctive procedure in addressing lesser digital deformities, the Weil osteotomy provides excellent results with few complications.

METATARSAL HEAD RESECTION

In cases of severe fixed deformity, degenerative arthritis at the MTPJ level, or after failed prior surgery, a partial or total metatarsal head resection may be warranted (**Fig. 10**). Originally described by DuVries,[11] a partial metatarsal head resection can successfully decompress the joint, realign the digit, and alleviate the pain. The main disadvantages of this procedure are increased stiffness at the MTPJ, recurrence of deformity, and transfer metatarsalgia.

Complete metatarsal head resection has been well documented in the rheumatoid patient population.[12] In cases of severe deformity and pain, this is an excellent procedure. Reize and colleagues[12] reviewed the results of panmetatarsal head resection in 34 patients with long-standing rheumatoid arthritis at a mean follow-up of 5.3 years. Overall, the patients rated their cosmetic and functional results as good. Most of

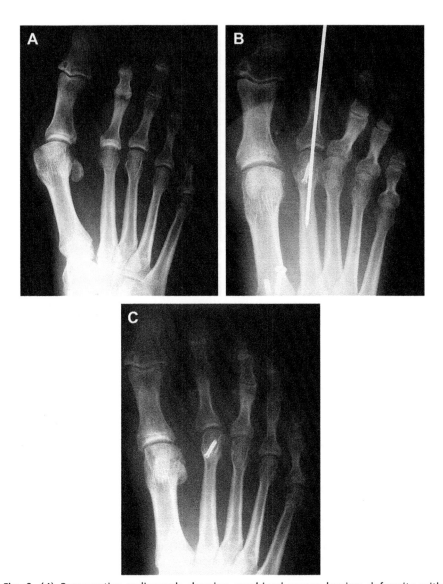

Fig. 9. (*A*) Preoperative radiograph showing combined severe bunion deformity with hammer toes and lesser MTPJ subluxation. (*B*) Early postoperative radiograph showing restored architecture to the forefoot. (*C*) Final radiograph shows that some medial deviation at the second MTPJ is present. Medial displacement of the Weil osteotomy might have offered an improved outcome, which could be observed in radiographically.

the patients (78%) were satisfied with reservations. The investigators rated the anatomic appearance (cosmesis) as good in 90% of the patients. However, the long-term results of this procedure are questionable. Hulse and Thomas[13] reviewed the results of 29 patients who underwent panmetatarsal head resection for rheumatoid forefoot deformities. At a mean follow-up of 6.57 years, pain ranged from nil to mild in 73% of the patients. The investigators did note a 17% reoperation rate of the resected

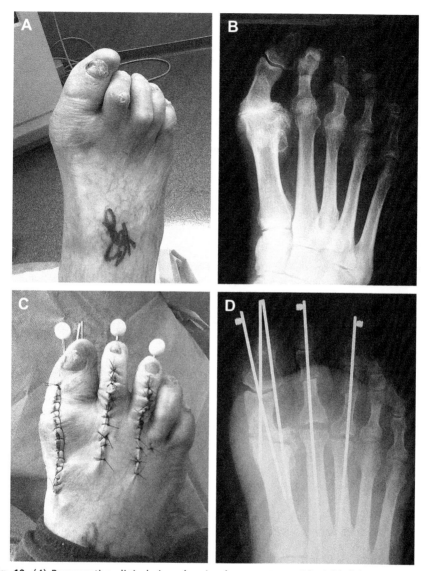

Fig. 10. (*A*) Preoperative clinical view showing hammer toes with rigid dislocation at the MTPJ. (*B*) Preoperative radiograph showing severe dislocation at lesser MTPJ level. (*C*) Immediate postoperative status with digits in corrected position. It is important to release the tourniquet in this type of procedure to assess for vascular compromise. (*D*) Postoperative radiograph showing metatarsal head resection.

metatarsal heads because of recurrence of pain and development of hypertrophic bone formation.

When performed on an isolated digit, the incisional approach is typically dorsal, centered over the affected metatarsal head. The metatarsal head is resected using a power saw. Although the metatarsal head may be resected using hand instrumentation, this can lead to spicule or shard formation, which may be difficult to remove. Once adequate resection has been performed, the MTPJ should be stabilized with

Kirschner wires. The patients may fully bear weight as tolerated in a surgical shoe. The Kirschner wires are typically left in place across the MTPJ for 4 to 6 weeks. When performing this procedure, careful inspection of the adjacent metatarsal level is necessary to avoid potential of transfer lesions or metatarsalgia.

AMPUTATION

For a severely deformed digit, amputation of the digit is generally considered a last resort. Gallentine and DeOrio[14] found that amputation of the second toe in elderly patients is acceptable for painful severe hammer toe deformities. The morbidity associated with more advanced reconstruction was avoided. Patient satisfaction was high and complications were minimal. Drift of the hallux into valgus did not seem to be a clinical problem. Cosmetically, amputation can be surprisingly acceptable, especially when performed in patients with severe bunion deformity.

SUMMARY

Digital deformities continue to be a common ailment among many patients who present to foot and ankle specialists. When conservative treatment fails to eliminate patient complaints, surgical correction remains a viable treatment option. With continued advances in fixation technology and techniques, surgeons continue to have better options for the achievement of excellent digital surgery outcomes.

REFERENCES

1. Coughlin MJ, Dorris J, Polk E. Operative repair of the fixed hammertoe deformity. Foot Ankle Int 2000;21(2):94–104.
2. Boyer ML, DeOrio JK. Transfer of the flexor digitorum longus for the correction of lesser toe deformities. Foot Ankle Int 2007;28(4):422–30.
3. Caterini R, Farsetti P, Tarantino U, et al. Arthrodesis of the toe joints with an intramedullary cannulated screw for correction of hammertoe deformity. Foot Ankle Int 2004;25(4):256–61.
4. Konkel KF, Menger AG, Retzlaff SA. Hammer toe correction using an absorbable intramedullary pin. Foot Ankle Int 2007;28(8):916–20.
5. Myerson MS, Jung HG. The role of toe flexor-to-extensor transfer in correcting metatarsophalangeal joint instability of the second toe. Foot Ankle Int 2005;26(9):675–9.
6. O'Kane C, Kilmartin T. Review of proximal interphalangeal joint excisional arthroplasty for the correction of second hammer toe deformity in 100 cases. Foot Ankle Int 2005;26(6):320–5.
7. Harmonson JK, Harkless LB. Operative procedures for the correction of hammertoe, claw toe, and mallet toe: a literature review. Clin Podiatr Med Surg 1996;13(2):211–20.
8. Roukis TS. A 1-piece shape-metal nitinol intramedullary internal fixation device for arthrodesis of the proximal interphalangeal joint in neuropathic patients with diabetes. Foot Ankle Spec 2009;2(3):130–4.
9. Choudhary RK, Theruvil B, Taylor GR. First metatarsophalangeal joint arthrodesis: a new technique of internal fixation by using memory compression staples. J Foot Ankle Surg 2004;43(5):312–7.
10. O'Kane C, Kilmartin TE. The surgical management of central metatarsalgia. Foot Ankle Int 2002;23(5):415–9.

11. DuVries HL. Disorders of the skin. In: Surgery of the foot. 2nd edition. St Louis (MO): Mosby; 1965. p. 168–9.
12. Reize P, Leichtle CI, Leichtle UG, et al. Long-term results after metatarsal head resection in the treatment of rheumatoid arthritis. Foot Ankle Int 2006;27(8): 586–90.
13. Hulse N, Thomas AM. Metatarsal head resection in the rheumatoid foot: 5-year follow-up with and without resection of the first metatarsal head. J Foot Ankle Surg 2006;45(2):107–12.
14. Gallentine JW, DeOrio JK. Removal of the second toe for severe hammertoe deformity in elderly patients. Foot Ankle Int 2005;26(5):353–8.

Metatarsal Fractures

Donald E. Buddecke, DPM[a],*, Matthew A. Polk, DPM[b],
Eric A. Barp, DPM[c]

KEYWORDS

• Metatarsal • Fracture • Jones • Injury

Acute metatarsal fractures represent a common cause of forefoot pain, accounting for 35% of all foot fractures and 5% of total skeletal fractures.[1] These fractures may occur as an isolated injury, concurrently with fractures of additional metatarsals, or in conjunction with Lisfranc injuries. Both direct and indirect traumas have been implicated in metatarsal fractures. Although most metatarsal fractures are a result of low-energy trauma,[2] high-energy crush injuries do occur with some frequency. As with other high-energy fractures, the soft tissue envelope becomes the primary concern (**Fig. 1**). These crush injuries need to be evaluated for compartment syndrome, and definitive treatment of the osseous component is delayed until the pressures are addressed. The recovery and condition of the soft tissue envelope then dictates when the definitive treatment is performed.

Metatarsal fractures can occur at any location on the bone and are generally divided by the region of occurrence into proximal metaphyseal (**Fig. 2**), diaphyseal or shaft (**Fig. 3**), and head and neck fractures (**Fig. 4**). Proximal metaphyseal and metatarsal base fractures may be associated with Lisfranc dislocations. These fractures often stay relatively well aligned because of the numerous articulations and soft tissue attachments.[2–4] Diaphyseal fractures are often oblique but may present in several fracture patterns. These fractures should be evaluated for shortening, angulation, and displacement.[5] In addition, stress fractures can progress to complete transverse fractures, and subsequent angulation or translation is a concern (**Fig. 5**). Distal metaphyseal fractures are commonly transverse or oblique, and if displacement is present, it typically occurs plantarly and laterally.[6] Because of the unique function of the first and fifth rays and the commonality between the central metatarsals, it is useful to examine metatarsal fractures in these separate components: first metatarsal, central metatarsals (including second, third, and fourth), and fifth metatarsal.

[a] Private Practice, 10780 V Street, Omaha, NE 68127, USA
[b] Saint Joseph Hospital, 2900 North Lakeshore Drive, Chicago, IL 60657, USA
[c] Private Practice, 5950 University Avenue, Suite 160, West Des Moines, IA 50266, USA
* Corresponding author.
E-mail address: debuddecke@yahoo.com

Clin Podiatr Med Surg 27 (2010) 601–624
doi:10.1016/j.cpm.2010.07.001
0891-8422/10/$ – see front matter © 2010 Elsevier Inc. All rights reserved.

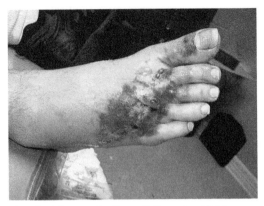

Fig. 1. Crush injury, showing damage to the soft tissue envelope.

FIRST METATARSAL

The importance of the first metatarsal and first ray has been previously reported.[7–10]

A traumatic disruption of the function or integrity of the first metatarsal can disturb the normal gait and cause pain at the first metatarsophalangeal joint, proximally along the medial column, or at the lesser metatarsals,[3,11] which can also lead to gait disturbances that can affect the entire limb.

The first metatarsal is the thickest, strongest, shortest, and heaviest of the metatarsal bones and has been reported to be the least frequently fractured metatarsal in adults, with an incidence of 1.5% of all metatarsal fractures.[1,11] However, a higher rate of fracture of the first metatarsal has been noted in pediatric populations,

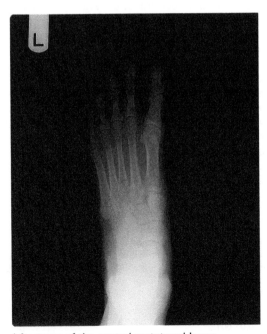

Fig. 2. Nondisplaced fractures of the central metatarsal bases.

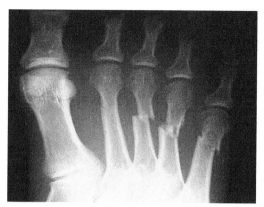

Fig. 3. Diaphyseal fractures of the second to fifth metatarsals.

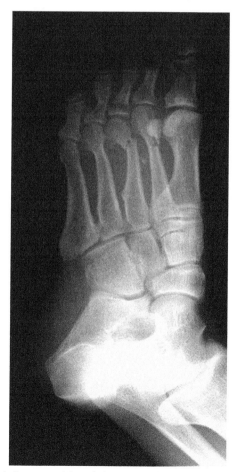

Fig. 4. Metatarsal neck fracture with malalignment of the third metatarsal. Also noted are fractures of the second metatarsal shaft and proximal phalanx of the third toe.

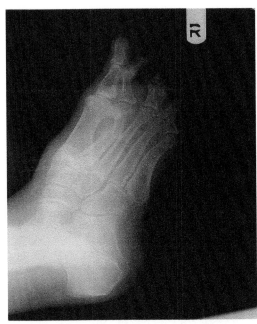

Fig. 5. Stress fracture of the second metatarsal that has progressed to complete fracture with malalignment.

especially in children younger than 5 years, whose injuries are more likely to have resulted from a fall from a height.[12]

Anatomically, the posterior aspect of the first metatarsal is large and concave, with a large kidney-shaped articular surface for its articulation with the medial cuneiform. The head of the first metatarsal is completely covered by articular cartilage for articulation with the proximal phalanx distally and the sesamoids plantarly. The first metatarsal motion is independent of the other metatarsals, allowing adaptability to uneven surfaces and ability to work in conjunction with hindfoot motion and variability. The first metatarsal is supplied by the dorsal metatarsal artery, the first plantar metatarsal artery, and the superficial branch of the medial plantar artery. The nutrient artery enters laterally in the distal one-third of the metatarsal, most often originating from the first dorsal artery.[3,11]

In the normal foot, there is equal distribution of weight across 6 different anatomic locations of the forefoot. Each of the lesser metatarsal heads along with the 2 sesamoids accommodates one-sixth of the weight during normal gait.[13] The importance of the first metatarsal is noted with its need to accommodate more pressure than the other metatarsals. Morton[10] noted that the axes of the forefoot were in balance when half of the weight passed through the first and second metatarsals and the other half of the weight passed through the third, fourth, and fifth metatarsals. Any disruption of this balance can lead to a dysfunctional foot.

The most frequent mechanism of injury of the first metatarsal in adults is either a standing fall or a direct blow, with the fracture most likely occurring in the diaphysis of the bone.[2] Twisting injuries, related to falls, occur when the foot is fixed on the ground and a sharp turn produces a mediolateral torque, which fractures the metatarsal. Axial loads may also cause a fracture by impacting the metatarsal into the medial cuneiform.[3,11] Direct crush injuries have been noted to be common in industry and often produce open fractures.[14] Avulsion fractures may occur at the first metatarsal base with plantar flexion and inversion type injuries because of the attachments of the peroneus longus and tibialis anterior at this level.[3,11]

CENTRAL METATARSALS

Central metatarsal fractures occur much more frequently than first metatarsal fractures and are more likely to affect multiple metatarsals. It has been reported that 63% of third metatarsal fractures occurred concurrently with second or fourth metatarsal fractures and 28% with both.[2] Petrisor and colleagues[2] also noted that all cases of multiple metatarsal fractures occurred in contiguous bones, so a careful radiographic examination is warranted when an isolated metatarsal fracture is encountered.

The central metatarsal bases bear joint surfaces for articulation with the tarsal bones. The second metatarsal articulates with all 3 cuneiform bones and is additionally stabilized by the Lisfranc ligament, which runs between the medial cuneiform and the base of the second metatarsal. The remaining metatarsal bases are joined by strong ligamentous support, both dorsally and plantarly. No similar structure unites the first and second metatarsals, allowing the first metatarsal its independent motion.

As previously mentioned, the bases of the central metatarsals are also stabilized by plantar, dorsal, and interosseous ligaments. Slips from the tibialis posterior represent the only extrinsic attachment. The metatarsal shafts are the origin for the intrinsic plantar and dorsal interossei.[1] The primary nutrient artery of the central metatarsals enters laterally, approximately 3.1 cm from the distal articular cartilage.[15]

Central metatarsal fractures are caused by indirect torsional trauma or direct trauma, with most fractures being attributed to the latter.[1,2] Direct trauma includes crushing blows to the dorsum of the foot or penetrating injuries (ie, gunshot wounds). Indirectly, a spiral or oblique fracture may be produced by a twisting injury over a fixed forefoot. Because of the relative lack of motion, soft tissue attachments, and stable proximal articulations, these fractures have a level of intrinsic stability. However, when displacement occurs, the central metatarsals are more likely to displace as a unit.[1,2]

FIFTH METATARSAL

The fifth metatarsal is the most frequently fractured, with a reported rate of up to 68% of all metatarsal fractures.[1] Similar to the first metatarsal, the fifth metatarsal functions with motion independent of the central metatarsals. The fifth metatarsal is also unique in that it has a proximal tuberosity for the insertion of the peroneus brevis tendon and the lateral slip of the plantar fascia. The tendon of the peroneus tertius also inserts into the dorsal aspect of the shaft. The fifth metatarsal base articulates with the cuboid proximally and with the fourth metatarsal base medially, with strong ligamentous attachments to both. The flexor digiti minimi and dorsal and plantar interossei originate from the fifth metatarsal.[16–19] Vascularity is provided by the dorsal metatarsal, the plantar metatarsal, and the fibular plantar marginal arteries. Investigations into the vascular supply of the fifth metatarsal indicate a poor blood supply to the proximal diaphysis, which may be associated with poor healing of fractures in this area.[17,20,21]

Fractures of the fifth metatarsal have a much greater emphasis on the anatomic location. Fifth metatarsal fractures are classified into head and neck fractures, shaft fractures, and fractures occurring at the base. Metatarsal neck fractures can be transverse, spiral, or impaction fractures (**Fig. 6**). Most fractures maintain an acceptable

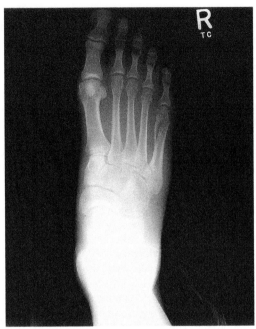

Fig. 6. Fracture of the fifth metatarsal neck with extension into the diaphyseal portion of bone.

alignment, but excessive sagittal plane displacement should be addressed because of weight-bearing considerations. Metatarsal shaft fractures are typically spiral. These fractures often have an associated butterfly fragment but can also present with significant comminution (**Fig. 7**). Comminuted fractures are usually related to direct impact or less-than-optimal bone quality. Both metatarsal neck and shaft fractures should also be evaluated for shortening.[16–18]

Fractures occurring at the base of the fifth metatarsal are of biggest concern because of the high incidence of tuberosity avulsion fractures and the controversy regarding fractures of the metaphyseal-diaphyseal junction. The fifth metatarsal avulsion fracture may be intra-articular (**Fig. 8**) or extra-articular. Traditionally, the avulsion fracture was thought to be caused by a violent contracture of the peroneus brevis tendon, but recent findings have implicated the lateral band of the plantar aponeurosis (**Fig. 9**) as the cause of the fracture.[22] It is likely that both structures can be implicated in isolation or in combination. At any rate, the mechanism is an inversion type of injury. Possible differential diagnoses of fifth metatarsal avulsion fractures include the presence of an apophysis in children and os peroneum or os vesalianum in adults, which is usually not difficult to determine based on clinical examination.

In addition to avulsion fractures, fifth metatarsal base fractures are further divided into acute (**Fig. 10**) metaphyseal-diaphysealfractures (Jones fractures) and proximal diaphyseal stress fractures. Fractures occurring distal to the fifth metatarsal base at the metaphyseal-diaphyseal junction are typically referred to as the Jones fractures. These fractures can be difficult to distinguish from the proximal diaphyseal stress fractures that occur in the same area. The differentiating factors include the acute injury causing the Jones fractures versus the existence of prodromal symptoms in stress fractures. Occasionally, the development of an acute-on-chronic injury occurs. This

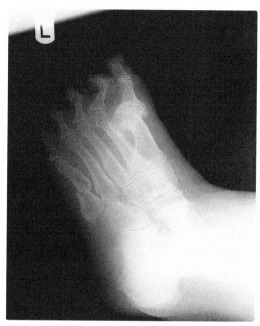

Fig. 7. Fracture of the fifth metatarsal shaft with associated comminution.

injury is seen in the presence of prodromal symptoms, but then a specific traumatic injury is reported by the patient. In this scenario, it is likely that the stress reaction or stress fracture was developing and the acute injury allowed the fracture to occur. The radiographic appearance can reveal signs of a chronic fracture/stress fracture despite the acute injury (**Fig. 11**).

These junctional fractures of the fifth metatarsal were further detailed by Torg and colleagues[23] These investigators studied 46 junctional fractures and divided them into acute fractures (those with a narrow fracture line and absence of medullary sclerosis), fractures with delayed union (those with widening of the fracture line and some

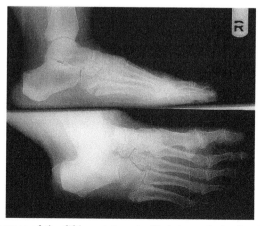

Fig. 8. Avulsion fracture of the fifth metatarsal with intra-articular involvement.

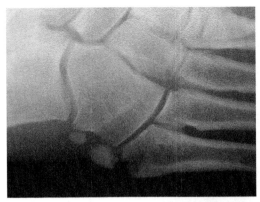

Fig. 9. Avulsion fracture of the fifth metatarsal base with displacement. This fracture was likely caused by pull of the lateral band of the plantar aponeurosis as opposed to that of the peroneus brevis, which would usually involve a larger fracture fragment because of the expansive attachment of this tendon.

evidence of medullary sclerosis), and fractures with nonunion (those with complete obliteration of the medullary canal by sclerotic bone).[23]

The acute junctional fracture was initially described in 1902.[24] Later, Stewart[25] discussed the decreased healing potential of these fractures and developed a classification system for describing the proximal fifth metatarsal fractures. He defined the Jones fracture as a transverse fracture at the metaphyseal-diaphyseal junction.[25] The cause

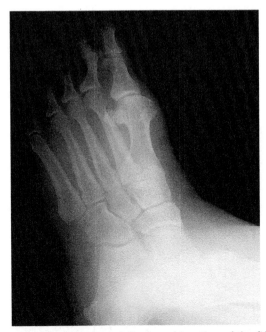

Fig. 10. Acute fracture at the metaphyseal-diaphyseal junction of the fifth metatarsal base (Jones fracture).

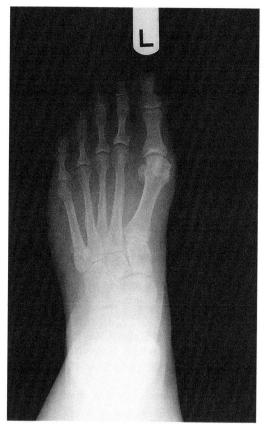

Fig. 11. This patient presented with an acute presentation after a traumatic event. However, radiographs reveal evidence of bony callus formation, suggesting previous injury or stress fracture. After specific questioning of the patient, there was evidence of prodromal symptoms even before the injury.

of this fracture is thought to be a large adduction force applied to the forefoot while the ankle is plantar flexed. The fracture site corresponds to the area between the insertion of the peroneus tertius and peroneus brevis tendons. Hindfoot varus has been identified as a possible predisposing factor to Jones fractures.[16,17,24,25] A varus attitude of the calcaneus certainly predisposes the lateral column of the foot to increased force, making it a contributing factor in stress fractures of the fifth metatarsal and, on occasion, the fourth metatarsal (**Fig. 12**).

TREATMENT
First Metatarsal Fractures

Strict attention to detail must be maintained in addressing the first metatarsal fractures because significant forces exist through the first metatarsal during gait. Any considerable displacement may have detrimental effects on the hallux through the metatarsophalangeal joint, causing gait abnormalities. Misalignment in the sagittal plane may limit the dorsiflexory/plantarflexory motion through the joint, causing traumatically induced hallux limitus/rigidus. Any sagittal plane malalignment is likely to lead to

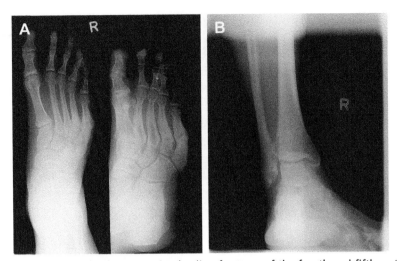

Fig. 12. (*A*) Radiographs demonstrating healing fractures of the fourth and fifth metatarsals. Associated metatarsus adductus deformity can be noted. (*B*) Mortise radiograph of the same patient demonstrating the varus attitude of the calcaneus placing an increased pressure on the lateral column of the foot.

metatarsalgia (**Fig. 13**). In addition, the hindfoot tries to compensate for this malalignment, often leading to additional foot or limb dysfunction. Significant displacement in the transverse plane may have the undesired effects of hallux valgus or varus. Frontal plane deformities are rare. Additional malalignment that often leads to a dysfunctional foot is shortening of the first metatarsal. Any loss of length needs to be restored to maintain the normal metatarsal parabola.

Criteria for surgical management of the fracture depend on the stability of the fracture. Anatomically, there is no ligamentous support from the first metatarsal to the lesser metatarsals. Fractures that display instability and displacement warrant surgical intervention. Nondisplaced fractures may be treated as per surgeon preference. Most of the literature supports a period of non–weight bearing in either a cast or a CAM boot

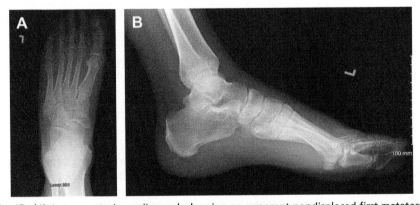

Fig. 13. (*A*) Anteroposterior radiograph showing an apparent nondisplaced first metatarsal shaft fracture. (*B*) Lateral radiograph of the same patient indicating plantar flexion of the distal portion of the first metatarsal.

for at least 2 to 3 weeks, with protective weight bearing to follow until radiographic evidence of healing is noted.[26,27] Truly nondisplaced fractures of the first metatarsal are rare, and close radiographic follow-up is necessary to ensure that alignment is maintained throughout the conservative therapy. Because of the force required to cause a fracture of this bone and the relative lack of stabilizing structures some displacement and malalignment is usually encountered.

Techniques for fixation of the first metatarsal depend on the fracture pattern. For diaphyseal fractures, buttress plating with screw fixation is the standard of care. The goals of internal fixation are to allow good bony apposition while restoring the osseous architecture. Strict attention to the length of the metatarsal, sesamoid apparatus, anatomic features of the metatarsophalangeal and tarsometatarsal joints, and planar alignment is paramount. Fixation of the fracture on the medial aspect may be done to protect the extensor tendons dorsally. The ideal position of plate fixation would be on the plantar aspect because this is the tension side of the fracture. However, dorsal or medial plate fixation is more common because of dissection restraints.

If there is significant comminution of the first metatarsal that would not support internal fixation, external fixation is warranted. The goal is to maintain the length of the first metatarsal to prevent transfer metatarsalgia. Patients with injuries involving severe comminution typically have damage to the soft tissue envelope as well. The application of external fixation is an option to protect the soft tissue envelope while maintaining stability of the fracture, further aiding in soft tissue repair. External fixation can span the first metatarsophalangeal joint and/or the first tarsometatarsal joint as deemed necessary for strength. This joint-spanning technique can also be used with plate fixation. The typical scenario is a comminuted fracture at the metatarsal base in which solid fixation cannot be accomplished. Surgeon's discretion dictates when joint-spanning techniques are to be used.

Management of intra-articular first metatarsal head fractures should attempt to preserve the integrity of the joint. If any joint incongruity is noted, open reduction with internal stabilization is mandated for a positive functional outcome. For metatarsal head fractures with significant impaction, cancellous bone grafting may be used. In isolated cases of significant comminution, primary metatarsophalangeal joint arthrodesis may be considered. Such cases are not commonly encountered.

Complications after first metatarsal fractures can include malunion, nonunion, and posttraumatic arthrosis. As mentioned previously, malunion can lead to not only local problems but also problems with dysfunction of the forefoot, midfoot, hindfoot, ankle, or entire limb. Nonunion after a first metatarsal fracture is not common. The healing potential is high because of the large percentage of cancellous bone relative to diaphyseal bone. Similar to other fractures involving joints, the incidence of arthrosis depends on the amount of damage at the time of injury and the quality of reduction of joint surfaces.

Central Metatarsal Fractures

As with almost all other fractures, nondisplaced or minimally displaced fractures of the central metatarsals are amenable to nonoperative treatment, including protected mobilization or immobilization in a cast, CAM boot, or even stiff-soled shoe. Acceptable levels of displacement or angulation of fractures vary depending on the treating physician. Although no definitive study is available to guide the decision making with regard to displacement or angulation, commonly acceptable levels have been reported to be less than 10° of angulation[13,28] and only 3 or 4 mm of translation in any plane.[29,30] Displacement in the sagittal plane is the least tolerated and can lead to excessive pressure if the fracture is plantarly displaced or angulated. Also, dorsally angulated fractures can cause dorsal or transfer irritation plantarly at the adjacent metatarsals. Transverse plane malalignment is better tolerated but can cause irritation as well. Close abutment of the metatarsal heads can lead to irritation with ambulation or even cause an intermetatarsal neuroma. Frontal plane malalignment is typically not a concern. The attachments between the metatarsal heads make frontal plane displacement an uncommon finding.

The goal of treatment is to maintain a functional forefoot. Specific details that should be considered for healing to take place include the metatarsal parabola, the sagittal plane position of the metatarsal heads, and bone-to-bone contact (**Fig. 14**). Closed manipulation of fractures of the central metatarsals can be accomplished with distal traction. However, one should be prepared to proceed with open reduction because maintaining the reduction with a closed means in a fracture with significant displacement is often an exercise of futility. In patients with significant comorbidities or vascular compromise, attempts are certainly warranted. In addition, the surgeon should be prepared for percutaneous pinning in cases in which reduction can be difficult to maintain.

Percutaneous Kirschner (K)-wire pinning can be performed with a variety of techniques. A common method is intramedullary pinning through the corresponding metatarsal head, which is usually done with a single K-wire fixation down the medullary canal, crossing the fracture site, and occasionally crossing the tarsometatarsal articulation when additional stability is deemed necessary. Additional K wires can be used for added strength but are rarely necessary. With multiple metatarsal fractures, the most displaced fracture is reduced and stabilized, often leading to anatomic, or near anatomic, restoration of the adjacent metatarsal fractures and eliminating the need for further fixation (**Fig. 15**). If displacement is maintained, additional manipulation can be performed followed by additional pinning. Alternative percutaneous pinning options have been described, including transverse pinning of the metatarsal heads.[31] Advantages of percutaneous pinning include the ability to maintain vascularity to the fractured bone. No extensive dissection is used, and subsequently, the soft tissue envelope is not disrupted. The main disadvantage is the inability for direct visualization and manipulation of the fracture. Thus, these advantages and disadvantages need to be weighed for each fracture.

When manipulation is not successful with closed means, open procedures are performed. Minimally invasive options are available depending on the fracture attitude. The theoretical advantage to the minimally invasive approach is the ability for direct visualization and manipulation of the fracture without extensive soft tissue stripping. A small incision can be placed over the fracture site to allow this visualization and manipulation. The distal fragment is then plantar flexed, giving access for insertion of the K wire down the medullary canal, which is then advanced distally through the metatarsal head. The toe is dorsiflexed, allowing the K wire to exit plantarly. A slightly modified technique has been described, which includes pinning across the proximal phalanx and exiting plantar to this bone.[13] The fracture is then reduced, and the K wire retrograded back across the fracture site, thus providing stability. The drawback, as with the percutaneous intramedullary fixation described earlier, is some disruption of the metatarsophalangeal joint and the potential for injury to the flexor tendons. However, it is unknown if this drawback has any long-term ill effect on the patient.

Standard open reduction with internal fixation is also an option for the treatment of central metatarsal fractures. This procedure has the advantage of direct visualization of the fracture, and thus, complete anatomic reduction should be easier. In addition, this procedure allows for more stable fixation options. However, this approach does

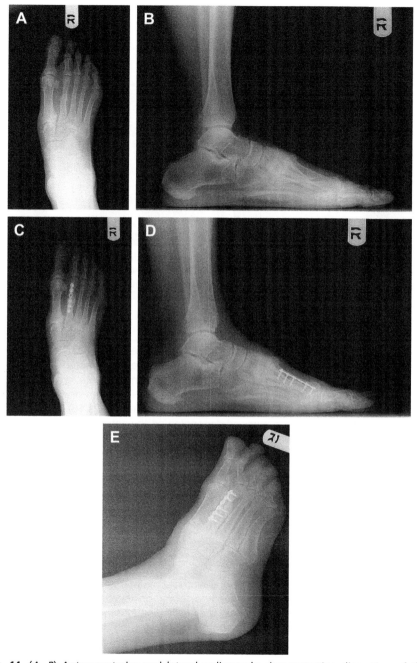

Fig. 14. (*A, B*) Anteroposterior and lateral radiographs demonstrating disruption of the metatarsal parabola with shortening of the second metatarsal and sagittal plane malalignment. Arthrosis is present at the first tarsometatarsal joint. This arthrosis led to the forefoot dysfunction and was the cause of the second metatarsal fracture. (*C–E*) Radiographs demonstrating reestablishment of the metatarsal parabola and realignment of the fracture in the sagittal plane. Although the first tarsometatarsal joint arthrosisand the fact that it was the cause of the second metatarsal stress fracture were discussed with the patient, the patient refused treatment of this joint.

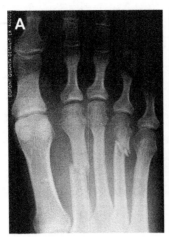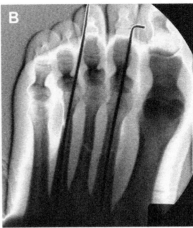

Fig. 15. (A) Shaft fractures of the central metatarsals. The maintenance of alignment of the third metatarsal can be noted. (B) K-wire fixation of the second and fourth metatarsals, showing complete reduction of the fractures and continued alignment of the third metatarsal.

lead to the disruption of more of the soft tissue envelope, even with the most meticulous dissection. Oblique or spiral oblique fractures may be amenable to interfragmentary screw fixation, which is often difficult in central metatarsal fractures because of the adjacent metatarsal making it difficult to manipulate instrumentation in the proper plane. More commonly, dorsal plate fixation is used. Minifragment or small fragment plates can be used, depending on the size of the metatarsal (**Fig. 16**). Locking plate constructs may also serve the purpose depending on the patient's condition.

Complications are uncommon. The most common complication after closed treatment of central metatarsal fractures includes metatarsalgia secondary to malunion and parabola disruption. A delayed union may be encountered, but nonunion is rarely a concern, which the authors think is because of the inherent stability noted within the central metatarsals as well as the musculature surrounding these bones adding to the abundance of vascularity available to promote healing. When a nonunion is noted in a central metatarsal fracture, it is typically the result of a long-standing stress fracture (and subsequently a mechanical problem) and not an acute injury.

Fifth Metatarsal Fractures

As noted earlier, the most commonly encountered metatarsal fracture is that of the fifth metatarsal. More specifically, the most common location of fracture of this bone is at the base. There exists controversy regarding treatment of fractures in this location. There has been an extensive amount of research regarding treatment of the fifth metatarsal base fracture, with most reports being written about the Jones fracture.[24,25,32–49]

There is controversy regarding the treatment of Jones fractures because of the difference in recommendations in various patient populations. It has been common to recommend surgical treatment of the Jones fracture in elite athletic populations. Conversely, a recommendation toward more conservative treatment is typically offered to others. However, a trend is developing toward recommending surgical intervention not only for elite athletes but also for other active populations and in cases in which a long period of immobilization is not desirable.

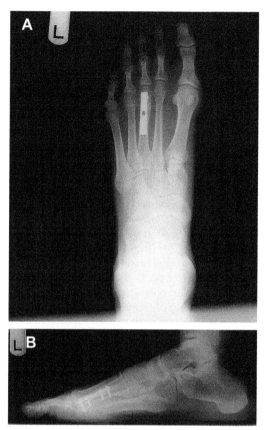

Fig. 16. (*A, B*) Anteroposterior and lateral radiographs depicting standard plate fixation of a third metatarsal shaft fracture.

Jones fractures are notorious for a tendency toward slow healing.[24,33–38] Several factors have been implicated for this delay. First, the nutrient artery enters at the medial aspect of this bone in close proximity to the fracture site.[20] Subsequently, this fracture has the potential to lead to at least a temporary disruption of this major blood supply.[21,35] Second, the metaphyseal-diaphyseal junction is already notorious for a limited vascular supply because of its location distal to the vascular-rich metaphyseal bone. Third, the base of the fifth metatarsal has strong ligamentous attachments to the cuboid and fourth metatarsal base. Because of these strong attachments, weight bearing at the metatarsal head causes the lever arm to transfer the forces to the area just distal to these attachments, which corresponds to the site of the fracture. As a result, the potential for motion is high with any weight-bearing activity, even in a fracture shoe or boot. This mechanical issue is the same reason that stress fractures occur in this area.

Conservative treatment of Jones fractures typically consists of protected mobilization in a CAM boot or even non–weight bearing for 6 to 8 weeks. An additional 6 to 8 weeks of normal weight-bearing activity is required before any exercise activity is implemented. Clinical assessment should reveal a lack of pain with direct palpation at the fracture site and signs of trabeculation crossing the fracture before implementing exercise activity. Computed tomographic (CT) evaluation may be a viable option before implementing athletic activity for high-level athletes to ensure complete heal-ing, likely decreasing the chance of refracture. However, with rising concerns of increased exposure to radiation, caution is recommended with the routine use of CT.

Numerous reports have demonstrated a tendency for delayed union, higher inci-dence of nonunion, and even refracture with closed treatment of these frac-tures.[23,38–40] In a randomized controlled clinical trial, Mologne and colleagues[39] demonstrated a significant difference when comparing early screw fixation with casting in acute Jones fractures. In this study, 18 patients were randomized to casting and 19 to intramedullary screw fixation. About 44% of the cast group were considered treatment failures, with 5 cases of nonunion, 1 of delayed union, and 2 of refracture. Only 1 of the 19 patients in the surgical group had a treatment failure (nonunion requiring bone grafting). In addition, the time to union and time to return to sport were almost twice as long in the cast group than in the surgical group.

Historically, surgical treatment of this junctional fracture was performed in the patients with delayed union or nonunion. Surgical treatment involved medullary curet-tage and inlay bone grafting. At present, the most common form of surgical treatment is intramedullary screw fixation.[39,41,42] This treatment is common for the acute frac-tures as well as for those with delayed union or nonunion. Bone grafting can still be performed when deemed necessary, such as in cases with complete medullary oblit-eration. Numerous reports have demonstrated decreased healing times, earlier return to activity, and less incidence of refracture after intramedullary screw fixation for these junctional fractures.[39,41–44] Konkel and colleagues[44] reported a 100% satisfaction rate and 98.5% union rate for all fifth metatarsal fractures (including 10 Jones fractures and 2 stress fractures) with only conservative treatment. These investigators, however, recommended "non-operative treatment of fifth metatarsal fractures for patients in whom the time to return to full activities is not critical."

Although intramedullary screw fixation is a common method of fixation, the size and type of screw to be used has been debated. Cannulated screws are commonly used because of the ease of application. The guidewire is easily advanced down the medul-lary canal, and its position confirmed with live fluoroscopy before screw placement. This procedure affords some adjustment in positioning before placement of the screw. However, there is some concern about the strength of cannulated screws versus solid screws. Reese and colleagues[45] compared cannulated titanium, cannulated stainless steel, and noncannulated stainless steel screws. They compared different types of 4-mm screws and the number of cycles to failure. The cannulated titanium screw failed after 4308 cycles, the cannulated stainless steel screw after 22,012 cycles, and the noncannulated screw after 44,523 cycles. This result showed an obvious increase in strength with the solid screw. These investigators also noted an increase in the number of cycles to failure with increasing screw size. Another study compared a solid screw developed specifically for Jones fracture fixation with other screws that were typically used for fixation of this fracture (Synthes 4.5-mm Malleolar screw [Synthes Inc, West Chester, PA, USA], Synthes 4.5-mm cannulated screw, and 4/5 Acutrak screw [Acumed Inc, Hillsboro, OR, USA]).[46] These investigators noted that the 4.5-mm Carolina screw (solid screw) (Wright Medical Technology Inc, Arlington, TN, USA) exceeded the other screws with regard to load cycles by 27-fold to 7067-fold, depending on the comparison.

Reports of screw failure have been documented after intramedullary screw fixation for Jones fractures.[33,47] Larson and colleagues[47] reported treatment failures in 6 of 15 patients who underwent intramedullary screw fixation, including 4 patients with refrac-ture and 2 with nonunion. Screw sizes used ranged from 4.0 to 6.5 mm. It was reported that 83% of the failures occurred in elite athletes. In addition, the mean time to return to activity was 6.8 weeks in the failure group compared with 9 weeks in the success group. Of the 6 failures, only 1 had radiographic confirmation of complete healing.

Refracture after intramedullary screw fixation has also been reported. Wright and colleagues[34] reported on 6 cases of refracture after intramedullary screw fixation with screws ranging from 4.0 to 5.0 mm. The study population that sustained the refracture included 4 professional football players, 1 collegiate basketball player, and 1 recreational athlete. Of the 6 refractures, 4 were in patients in whom cannulated screws were used. It would seem that this smaller size of screw is inappropriate for such a high-demand patient population.

The most appropriate size of screw has not yet been determined. Obviously, the larger-diameter screws will have greater resistance to failure. However, there is a limit to the size of screw that can be used based on the size of the medullary canal. Breakage of the metatarsal shaft has been reported with the use of 6.5-mm screws.[46,48,49] As a result, the authors' method for determining screw size is based on the results of preoperative radiographs. The medullary canal is measured on the anteroposterior, lateral, and oblique views, and the appropriate-sized screw is then used, which typically is a 4.5-, 5.0-, or 5.5-mm screw. Occasionally, a 4.0-mm screw is used in a smaller patient with less physical demands. Several other factors are taken into account when selecting the appropriate-sized screw, including the patient size and patient activity levels. If the size of the medullary canal allows only a smaller-sized screw (ie, 4.0 mm) and the patient is of larger size and/or is active athletically, the time before allowing a return to activity is increased. Also, a solid screw is typically preferred to a cannulated screw. Curvature of the fifth metatarsal needs to be considered as well. Screw length is optimal when all threads are distal to the fracture site and several threads are engaged in the inner cortices of the bone. Care should be taken to prevent penetration of the medial cortex with an excessively long screw. Although it is typically not difficult to have all threads distal to the fracture site with partially threaded screws, extremely curved metatarsals may make it difficult to prevent medial cortex penetration (**Fig. 17**). Individualized treatment is recommended.

Other surgical treatments have been described, including percutaneous pinning,[50] tension band wiring,[51] and external fixation.[52] Medullary curettage and bone grafting is used for nonunion,[23,36] which can be done with plate fixation or even in conjunction with intramedullary screw fixation (**Fig. 18**).

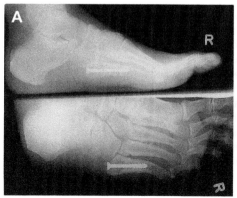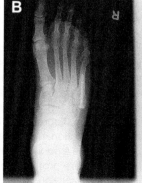

Fig. 17. (*A, B*) Intramedullary screw fixation of a Jones fracture. There is engagement of the dorsal cortex because of the curvature of the bone in the sagittal plane and the engagement of the medial cortex because of the curvature of the bone in the transverse plane.

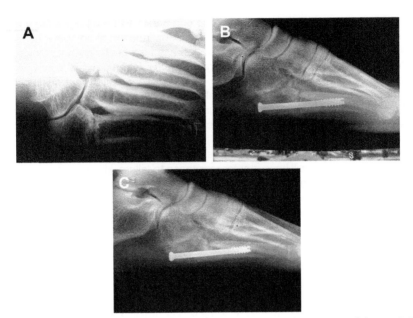

Fig. 18. (*A*) Nonunion of the fifth metatarsal as indicated by obliteration of the medullary canal. (*B*) Fifth metatarsal nonunion after medullary curettage, bone grafting, and intramedullary screw fixation. (*C*) Radiograph demonstrating complete healing of the previous nonunion site.

Other than the difficult healing potential of these fractures, complications are not common. One of the most common complications after intramedullary screw fixation of fifth metatarsals is hardware irritation from the screw head. The head of the screw can irritate the sural nerve, or the incision and scarring can lead to sural nerve complications. Other complications that are encountered are generally a direct result of the surgical technique, including improper placement of the screw, such as penetration of the medial cortex, or use of incorrect screw size.

The technique for intramedullary screw fixation includes making an incision proximal to the styloid process. If medullary curettage and bone grafting is needed, this incision can be lengthened. Otherwise, a small stab incision is made. The patient is positioned in a lateral decubital position with adequate room for fluoroscopy. The alignment of the guidewire can be assessed with fluoroscopy, and appropriate mapping performed. Ideally, the guidewire enters the styloid process slightly higher and slightly medial to the tip of the bone. The guidewire is then advanced down the medullary canal and assessed with fluoroscopy in various planes. It should be ensured that the guidewire is down the canal and does not exit any cortex. Once the guidewire placement is confirmed, the proximal cortex can be drilled and appropriate-length screw placed. Again, fluoroscopy is used to critically assess the position of fixation.

In contrast to junctional fractures of the fifth metatarsal, avulsion fractures of the styloid process have a good tendency to heal. Avulsion fractures are located in metaphyseal bone and are proximal to the mechanical forces that subject the junctional fracture to motion. Avulsion fractures are caused by an inversion type of injury, leading to pull of the peroneus brevis tendon and avulsion of the styloid process. A slip of the lateral band of the plantar fascia has also been implicated in causing avulsion fracture.[22] It was thought that the insertion site of the peroneus brevis was too expansile to cause many of the avulsion fractures that occur just at the tip of the styloid process. However, nondisplaced and minimally displaced fractures are successfully treated with immobilization in a weight-bearing CAM boot.

When displacement occurs, open reduction with internal fixation or percutaneous fixation is recommended. Fractures involving a small portion of the styloid process can be excised. The insertion site of the peroneus brevis is usually expansive enough that tendon anchoring is not necessary. However, larger fractures that are excised may mandate reattachment of the brevis tendon (**Fig. 19**). Fractures with more than 2 mm of displacement or those involving 30% or more of the joint should be considered for surgical intervention.[53,54] One of the more common methods of fixation includes intramedullary screw fixation as previously described for Jones fracture fixation. Similar to intramedullary screw fixation for Jones fractures, there is disagreement in the size of screw that is recommended. However, the technique is the same for fixation of this fracture pattern. Choosing the appropriate screw size and making sure to overdrill the fracture fragment prior to screw placement are important steps to prevent fracturing this fragment. Additional discussion of fixation of this fracture has been with regard to true intramedullary fixation versus fixation that engages the medial cortex (bicortical fixation) of the fifth metatarsal[55] and comparison of tension band fixation with bicortical screw fixation.[56] Morshirfar and colleagues[55] performed a cadaveric study comparing standard intramedullary screw fixation with lag screw fixation by engaging the medial cortex of the fifth metatarsal. They demonstrated a significantly greater load to failure in the lag screw technique than in the intramedullary screw technique. Caution should be taken with placement of screws across these avulsion fractures. Fracture of the fragment can occur, especially with larger screws and smaller fragments. Tension band fixation is also a common option for fixation of these fractures. This approach affords solid fixation with smaller pins in place of larger-diameter screws and risking fracture of the fragment.

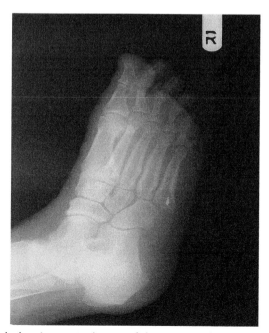

Fig. 19. Radiograph showing reattachment of the peroneus brevis tendon with soft tissue anchor after excision of the avulsion fracture of fifth metatarsal.

Fractures of the fifth metatarsal shaft are commonly encountered. The typical fracture pattern is spiral and may have a butterfly fragment or further comminution. Evaluation should be directed toward the amount of displacement and any angulation or shortening. Although disruption in length or position of the fifth metatarsal head is more easily tolerable than that of the other metatarsals, the goal should be to maintain as normal a metatarsal parabola as possible.

Conservative treatment is often successful and includes initial immobilization and non–weight bearing for 4 to 5 weeks followed by protected weight bearing in a fracture boot for an additional 4 weeks. Surgical intervention should be implemented when displacement is greater than 3 to 4 mm, when angulation is greater than 10°,[54] or if extensive shortening is noted. Fixation can be accomplished with interfragmentary screw fixation or plate fixation. Caution is warranted if interfragmentary fixation is planned. Often, there is a butterfly fragment, making stability difficult. In addition, the shaft of this bone can be relatively fragile, and interfragmentary fixation can cause further comminution. Consequently, the authors typically use plate fixation for many of these fifth metatarsal shaft fractures (**Fig. 20**).

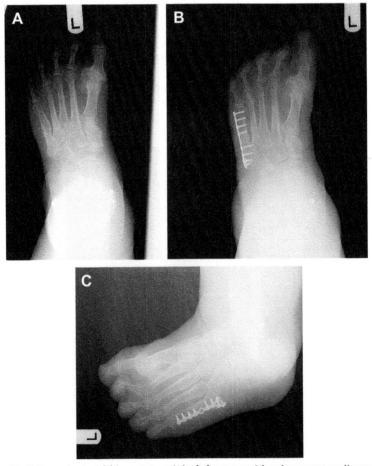

Fig. 20. (A–C) Comminuted fifth metatarsal shaft fracture with subsequent realignment and stabilization with locking plate construct.

The final fracture location noted within the fifth metatarsal is the neck fracture. This fracture is often relatively nondisplaced and amenable to healing with weight-bearing ambulation in a fracture boot. In cases with significant displacement, fixation is necessary. Similar to the techniques previously described, fixation can be done with percutaneous pinning or open reduction with pinning. Less commonly, plate fixation can be performed.

As with all fractures, delayed union, nonunion, and malunion are always possible when the integrity of the osseous segment has been disrupted. Delayed unions and nonunions lead to extended time away from activity and temporary change in lifestyle, which may lead to the need for surgical intervention or revision surgery. Malunion can cause transfer metatarsalgia and any other problem associated with metatarsal parabola disruption.

A less common issue noted with metatarsal fractures is arthritis. Most metatarsal fractures do not involve articulations. However, arthritis is a problem that the physician needs to be aware of with fractures involving the base or head of these bones.

Other complications can include those involving nerve structures around the forefoot. The issues with the sural nerve can be encountered with surgical intervention of any fifth metatarsal fracture. These issues are typically noted with incisions placed in the area of the nerve or with screw head irritation with intramedullary screw placement. Other superficial nerve issues can be encountered with surgical approaches to the other metatarsals. The branches from the cutaneous nerves are always at risk with dorsal incision placement in the forefoot. In addition, there is not a lot of soft tissue coverage in this area, making injury or entrapment a possible complication. Surgical technique becomes extremely important in this situation. Prevention of the problem is typically easier than later treatment of the complication.

SUMMARY

Metatarsal fractures can present with a variety of situations. Ranging from the relatively benign, isolated central metatarsal fracture to the crush injury leading to extensive damage of the soft tissue and osseous component, these fractures can cause a significant inconvenience to the patient. With the exception of the fifth metatarsal fractures, little standardization is available for the treatment of metatarsal fractures. Controversy still exists regarding to the proper treatment of various patient populations for junctional fifth metatarsal fractures. Consequently, the foot and ankle physician must understand the various attitudes that each fracture exhibits.

The importance of the first metatarsal with regard to overall foot function makes anatomic alignment paramount. Attention to detail can help prevent long-term sequelae. Central metatarsal fractures have a high chance of union, with little known about extensive complications. However, disruption in the metatarsal parabola can cause undue discomfort. The fifth metatarsal is by far the most common metatarsal that is fractured. A large percentage of this fracture is amenable to conservative treatment. When surgical intervention is implemented, the patient and surgeon can expect a good outcome.

REFERENCES

1. Urteaga A, Lynch M. Fractures of the central metatarsals. Clin Podiatr Med Surg 1995;12:759–62.
2. Petrisor B, Ekrol I, Court-Brown C. The epidemiology of metatarsal fractures. Foot Ankle Int 2006;27:172–5.

3. Maskill J, Bohay D, Anderson J. First ray injuries. Foot Ankle Clin N Am 2006;11: 143–63.
4. Pearson J. Fractures of the base of the metatarsals. BMJ 1962;1:1052–4.
5. Maxwell J. Open or closed treatment of metatarsal fractures: indications and techniques. J Am Podiatry Assoc 1983;73:100–6.
6. Heckman J. Fractures and dislocations of the foot. In: Rockwood C, Green D, editors. Fractures. 2nd edition. Philadelphia: JB Lippencott; 1984. p. 1808–9.
7. Christensen J, Jennings M. Normal and abnormal function of the 1st ray. Clin Podiatr Med Surg 2009;26(3):355–71.
8. Hicks J. The mechanics of the foot. Part I: the joints. J Anat 1953;87:345–57.
9. Root ML, Orien WP, Weed JH. Motion of the joints of the foot: the first ray. In: Clinical biomechanics. Normal and abnormal function of the foot, vol. II. Los Angeles; 1977. p. 46–51, 350–4.
10. Morton D. Dorsal hypermobility of the first metatarsal segment: part III. In: Morton DJ, editor. The human foot: its evolution, physiology, and functional disorders. New York: Columbia University; 1935. p. 187–95.
11. Saraiya M. First metatarsal fractures. Clin Podiatr Med Surg 1995;12:749–59.
12. Singer G, Cichocki M, Schalamon J, et al. A study of metatarsal fractures in children. J Bone Joint Surg Am 2008;90:772–6.
13. Hansen ST. Foot injuries. In: Browner BD, Jupiter JB, Levine AM, et al, editors. Skeletal trauma. Philadelphia: WB Saunders Company; 1998. p. 2405–38.
14. Johnson V. Treatment of fractures of the forefoot in industry. In: Bateman JB, editor. Foot science. Philadelphia: WB Saunders; 1976. p. 257.
15. Jaworek T. The intrinsic vascular supply to the first and lesser metatarsals: Surgical considerations. Chicago (IL): Sixth Annual Northlake Surgical Seminar; 1976.
16. McBryde A. The complicated jones fracture, including revision and malalignment. Foot Ankle Clin N Am 2009;14:151–68.
17. Landorf K. Clarifying proximal diaphyseal fifth metatarsal fractures: the acute fracture versus the stress fracture. J Am Podiatr Med Assoc 1999;89:398–404.
18. Vogler H, Westlin N, Mlodzienski A, et al. Fifth metatarsal fractures: biomechanics, classification and treatment. Clin Podiatr Med Surg 1995;12:725–47.
19. Chuckpaiwong B, Queen R, Easley M, et al. Distinguishing Jones and proximal diaphyseal fractures of the fifth metatarsal. Clin Orthop Relat Res 2008;466: 1966–70.
20. Shereff M, Yang Q, Kummer F. Vascular anatomy of the fifth metatarsal. Foot Ankle 1991;11:350–3.
21. Smith J, Arnoczky S, Hersh A. The intraosseous blood supply of the fifth metatarsal: implications for proximal fracture healing. Foot Ankle 1992;13:143.
22. Richli W, Rosenthal D. Avulsion fracture of the fifth metatarsal: experimental study of pathomechanics. AJR Am J Roentgenol 1984;143:889–91.
23. Torg J, Balduini F, Zelko R, et al. Fractures of the base of the fifth metatarsal distal to the tuberosity. Classification and guidelines for non-surgical and surgical management. J Bone Joint Surg Am 1984;66(2):209–14.
24. Jones R. Fracture of the base of the fifth metatarsal bone by indirect violence. Ann Surg 1902;35:103–11.
25. Stewart I. Jones's fracture: fracture of the base of the fifth metatarsal. Clin Orthop 1960;16:190–8.
26. LaPorta G. Fracture of the first metatarsal. In: Scurran BL, editor. Foot and ankle trauma. New York: Churchill Livingstone; 1989. p. 323–45.
27. Mann RA, Coughlin JM. Surgery of the foot and ankle. 6th edition. St. Louis (MO): Mosby Inc; 1993.

28. Early J. Metatarsal fractures. In: Bucholz R, Heckman J, Rockwood C, et al, editors. Rockwood and green's fractures in adults. Lippincott, Williams, & Wilkins; 2001. p. 2215.

29. Shereff M. Complex fractures of the metatarsals. Orthopedics 1990;13(8):875–82.

30. Armagan O, Shereff M. Injuries to the toes and metatarsals. Orthop Clin North Am 2001;32(1):1–10.

31. Donahue M, Manoli A. Technical tip: transverse percutaneous pinning of metatarsal neck fractures. Foot Ankle Int 2004;25(6):438–9.

32. DeLee J, Evans J, Julian J. Stress fracture of the fifth metatarsal. Am J Sports Med 1983;11(5):349–53.

33. Glasgow M, Naranja R, Glascow S, et al. Analysis of failed surgical management of fractures of the base of the fifth metatarsal distal to the tuberosity: the Jones fracture. Foot Ankle Int 1996;17(8):449–57.

34. Wright R, Fischer D, Shively R, et al. Refracture of proximal fifth metatarsal (Jones) fracture after intramedullary screw fixation in athletes. Am J Sports Med 2000;28(5):732–6.

35. Lawrence S, Botte M. Jones' fractures and related fractures of the proximal fifth metatarsal. Foot Ankle 1993;14(6):358–65.

36. Zelko R, Torg J, Rachun A. Proximal diaphyseal fractures of the fifth metatarsal—treatment of the fractures and their complications in athletes. Am J Sports Med 1979;7(2):95–101.

37. Zogby R, Baker B. A review of nonoperative treatment of Jones' fracture. Am J Sports Med 1987;15(4):304–7.

38. Dameron T. Fractures and anatomical variations of the proximal portion of the fifth metatarsal. J Bone Joint Surg Am 1975;57(6):788–92.

39. Mologne T, Lundeen J, Clapper M, et al. Early screw fixation versus casting in the treatment of acute Jones fractures. Am J Sports Med 2005;33(7):970–5.

40. Kavanaugh J, Brower T, Mann R. The Jones fracture revisited. J Bone Joint Surg Am 1978;60:776–82.

41. Porter D, Duncan M, Meyer S. Fifth metatarsal Jones fracture fixation with a 4.5-mm cannulated stainless steel screw in the competitive and recreational athlete: a clinical and radiographic evaluation. Am J Sports Med 2005;33(5): 726–33.

42. Porter D, Rund A, Dobslew R, et al. Comparison of 4.5-and 5.5-mm cannulated stainless steel screws for fifth metatarsal Jones Fracture fixation. Foot Ankle Int 2009;30(1):27–33.

43. Portland G, Kelikian A, Kodros S. Acute surgical management of Jones' fractures. Foot Ankle Int 2003;24(11):829–33.

44. Konkel K, Menger A, Retzlaff S. Nonoperative treatment of fifth metatarsal fractures in an orthopaedic suburban multispeciality practice. Foot Ankle Int 2005; 25(9):704–7.

45. Reese K, Litsky A, Kaeding C, et al. Cannulated screw fixation of Jones fractures. A clinical and biomechanical study. Am J Sports Med 2004;32:1736–42.

46. Nunley J, Glisson R. A new option for intramedullary fixation of Jones fractures: the charlotte Carolina Jones fracture system. Foot Ankle Int 2008;29:1216–21.

47. Larson C, Almekinders L, Taft T, et al. Intramedullary screw fixation of Jones fractures. Analysis of failure. Am J Sports Med 2002;30:55–60.

48. Horst F, Gilbert B, Glisson R, et al. Torque resistance after fixation of Jones fractures with intramedullary screws. Foot Ankle Int 2004;25:914–9.

49. Kelly I, Glisson R, Fink C, et al. Intramedullary screw fixation of Jones fractures. Foot Ankle Int 2001;22:585–9.

50. Arangio G. Transverse proximal diaphysial fracture of the fifth metatarsal: a review of 12 cases. Foot Ankle 1992;13(9):547–9.
51. Sarimo J, Rantanen J, Orava S, et al. Tension-band wiring for fractures of the fifth metatarsal located in the junction of the proximal metaphysic and diaphysis. Am J Sports Med 2006;34(3):476–80.
52. Lombardi C, Connolly F, Silhanek A. The use of external fixation for treatment of the acute Jones fracture: a retrospective review of 10 cases. J Foot Ankle Surg 2004;43(3):173–8.
53. Koslowsky T, Gausepohl T, Mader K, et al. Treatment of displaced proximal fifth metatarsal fractures using a new one-step fixation technique. J Trauma 2010; 68(1):122–5.
54. Zwitser E, Beederveld R. Fractures of fifth metatarsal: diagnosis and treatment. Injury 2009;41(6):555–62.
55. Moshirfar A, Campbell J, Molloy S, et al. Fifth metatarsal tuberosity fracture fixation: a biomechanical study. Foot Ankle Int 2003;24(8):630–3.
56. Husain Z, DeFronzo D. Relative stability of tension band versus two-cortex screw fixation for treating fifth metatarsal base avulsion fractures. J Foot Ankle Surg 2000;39(2):89–95.

Arthroplasty for Fifth Toe Deformity

Walter W. Strash, DPM

KEYWORDS

• Arthroplasty • Fifth toe • Hammertoe • Footgear

Fifth toe positional problems typically cause irritation with various forms of footgear.[1–3] The position of the toe causes irritation against the toe box of the shoe. There are 3 varieties of deformity, a cock-up deformity, a plantar flexion deformity, and an overlapping deformity, which occur at the fifth metatarsophalangeal joint of the fifth toe. Each deformity has different physical examination findings, causes, and treatment. With some deformities, conservative treatment can be successful in controlling a patient's discomfort. The cock-up deformity is most commonly seen in older patients. The typical presentation is a dorsiflexed and abducted fifth toe. The onset is usually slow and insidious, and patients typically do not seek treatment until they have difficulties with all forms of footgear, including pain and callus formation. The plantar flexed and overlapping deformities more commonly occur in younger age groups and are often congenital. The signs and symptoms of this deformity are similar to those of the cock-up deformity, and patients have difficulty with shoes fitting properly.

A corn (hyperkeratotic lesion) is often seen overlying the proximal interphalangeal joint of the fifth toe. Footwear is the often-cited cause because compression from the toe box creates irritation to the skin and an accumulation of hyperkeratotic tissue. With an abducted deformity, hyperkeratotic tissue can develop in the web space and become macerated creating a soft corn (heloma molle). This deformity often leads to infection because the moisture causes a breakdown of the skin and a portal for bacteria to enter the area.

PHYSICAL EXAMINATION

The metatarsal phalangeal joint may be contracted with the proximal portion of the fifth toe in a cock-up position. There may be a varus component to the position of the fifth toe. In younger patients, the joint is flexible and may be easily reducible. With time, the capsule and extensor mechanism become contracted, and the fifth toe becomes tighter and less reducible. Often there is a palpable callus on the proximal interphalangeal joint (**Fig. 1**).

Private Practice - Alamo Family Foot & Ankle Care, San Antonio, TX, USA
E-mail address: podcanuck@aol.com

Clin Podiatr Med Surg 27 (2010) 625–628
doi:10.1016/j.cpm.2010.08.001
0891-8422/10/$ – see front matter © 2010 Published by Elsevier Inc.

podiatric.theclinics.com

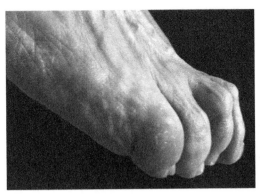

Fig. 1. Callus on the proximal interphalangeal joint.

With a plantar flexion deformity, the fifth toe is in a plantar flexed position and may be varus rotated. There is typically a flexion contracture of the flexor tendons of the fifth toe, and attempts at manually straightening the toe on examination are a challenge.

The overlapping deformity may be congenital. The fifth toe is contracted and rests on the dorsal side of the adjacent fourth toe. The congenital deformity is fixed and irreducible. Most patients relate to a history of having the problem for as long as they can remember. In the early developmental deformity, the fifth toe can be reduced manually and brought back into a neutral position. However, with time, the developmental deformity becomes more rigid and fixed.

Radiographic evaluation of the cock-up toe deformity shows the subluxation and dorsiflexion of the proximal phalanx on the head of the fifth metatarsal. A varus positioning of the proximal phalanx may be observed. There may also be a prominence or enlarged head of the proximal phalanx. In the case of the soft corn, an enlarged medial head of the proximal phalanx may be seen.

SOLUTIONS

From a nonsurgical standpoint, taping and strapping of the toes are usually unsuccessful. Strapping of the fifth toe in a corrected position by buddy splinting to the fourth toe only allows for temporary correction because once the strapping is removed, the fifth toe returns to its prior position. Shoes with a wider and deeper toe box along with padding of the fifth toe may offer the elderly and patients with reduced physical demands some relief. Along with the debridement of the soft corn, the use of lamb's wool and various soft toe spacer pads may reduce maceration to the interspace and provide patients with temporary relief.

STANDARD OR BASIC HAMMERTOE PROCEDURE

Resection of the head of the proximal phalanx of the fifth toe or fifth toe arthroplasty is a common, relatively simple, and effective procedure for painful lesions of the proximal interphalangeal joint. This procedure relieves the flexion contracture of the proximal interphalangeal joint and may need to be combined with extensor and capsular release over the metatarsal phalangeal joint if extensor contracture at the metatarsal phalangeal exists. Temporary pinning of the toe may also be necessary as an adjunct to the hammertoe repair.

Frontal plane rotation of the fifth toe can be accomplished with this procedure, and proper semielliptical skin incision placement over the proximal interphalangeal joint is helpful in obtaining both sagittal and frontal plane correction.

Most commonly, a dorsolinear incision is placed over the proximal interphalangeal joint. Alternatively, 2 semielliptical incisions may be made from proximal lateral to distal medial to aid in derotation and frontal plane correction. The hyperkeratotic lesion is excised within the skin wedge.

The incision is deepened through the superficial fascia to expose the capsule and extensor tendon. At the level of the proximal interphalangeal joint, a transverse incision is made proximally to the base of the middle phalanx, leaving a small portion of extensor tendon. The proximal interphalangeal joint capsule and collateral ligaments are carefully incised with a 64-blade because the use of this blade is helpful in preventing an inadvertent buttonholing.

The head of the proximal phalanx is now exposed and resected, using a small sagittal saw, with the amount of bone removed depending on the amount of flexion contracture at the proximal interphalangeal joint. The proximal phalangeal stump is then rasped smooth and the long extensor tendon is repaired. Stability of this repair is enhanced with the repair of the medial and lateral collateral ligaments to prevent the possibility of a flail toe (**Fig. 2**).

The fifth toe is then held in a rectus position as the sterile dressing is applied. Patients' feet are placed in a postoperative shoe for a 2-week period. After suture removal, further splinting of the fifth toe is helpful for an additional 2 to 3 weeks to support the soft tissues during healing and scar remodeling. This splinting aids in maintaining the corrected position of the fifth toe.

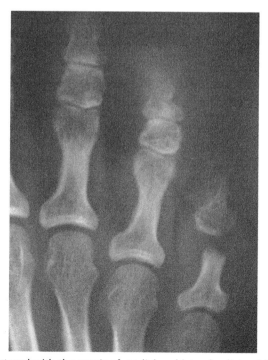

Fig. 2. Stability restored with the repair of medial and lateral collateral ligaments.

MANAGEMENT OF COMPLICATIONS

Shortening of the fifth toe occurs with the arthroplasty procedure, and instability manifests itself as a floppy toe. This complication is exaggerated if a large partial condylectomy is performed. Typically, there is no functional consequence other than the toe catching on socks. A solution to failed fifth toe arthroplasty is the application of a metal or Silastic lesser toe implant.

If the toe is undercorrected, recurrence may arise. Placement of the toe in a corrected position with postoperative bandages or Kirschner wire fixation is helpful. However, pin placement for 3 to 4 weeks cannot correct a soft tissue deformity that has not been addressed at the time of surgery.

The small area for the fifth toe arthroplasty requires protection of the neurovascular structures. Injury to a proper digital branch may lead to numbness of the toe. Preoperatively, the patient should be informed that the fifth toe will not have full function as a result of shortening and disruption of the extensor mechanism.

SUMMARY

Although there are variations on the fifth toe arthroplasty, such as the derotational procedure, Z-plasty, and V-Y skin plasty techniques, the standard or basic arthroplasty offers the simplest approach and can be used with most fifth hammertoes. The concept discussed in this article is not difficult to perform and master, requiring minimal preparation with a high rate of patient satisfaction.

REFERENCES

1. Root MC, Orien WP, Weed JH. Normal and abnormal function of the foot, clinical biomechanics. Los Angeles: Clinical Biomechanics Corporation; 1977. p. 457.
2. Dobbs BM. Arthroplasty of the fifth toe. Clin Podiatr Med Surg 1986;3(1):29–39.
3. Smith TF, Pfeifer KD. Surgical repair of fifth digit deformities. In: Banks AS, Downey MS, Martin DE, et al, editors. McGlamry's comprehensive textbook of foot & ankle surgery. Lippincott Williams & Wilkins; 2001. p. 311–7.

Current Concepts and Techniques in Foot and Ankle Surgery

Juxta-articular Osteoid Osteoma of the Talar Neck: A Case Report

Andreas F. Mavrogenis, MD[a],*, Rozalia Dimitriou, MD[a],
Ioannis S. Benetos, MD[b], Demetrios S. Korres, MD[b],
Panayiotis J. Papagelopoulos, MD, DSc[a]

KEYWORDS

• Juxta-articular osteoid osteoma • Ankle • Tumor • Foot pain

Juxta-articular osteoid osteomas are rare and tend to have an atypical presentation, including variable articular pain and symptoms related to intense or chronic synovitis, such as joint tenderness, soft tissue swelling, joint effusion, stiffness, and decreased range of motion, as with any monoarticular inflammatory arthropathy.[1–4] Unlike the more classically located extra-articular osteoid osteomas, clinical symptoms of juxta-articular osteoid osteomas are misleading.[2–7] The nidus commonly is identified on radiographs and bone scintigraphy may not show classical features.[1,2,5] The hip is the most common location of juxta-articular osteoid osteomas; the ankle, elbow, wrist, and knee joints are less commonly affected.[1,4,8–22]

Osteoid osteomas in the neck of the talus have proved a vexing diagnostic challenge.[8–22] This article presents a patient with a juxta-articular osteoid osteoma at the talar neck initially misdiagnosed as ankle sprain and anterior ankle impingement.

CASE REPORT

A 33-year-old man was admitted to the authors' institution with a 2-year history of right ankle pain. Initial diagnosis from the treating physicians included ankle sprain and anterior ankle impingement. He had painful restriction of motion of the left ankle joint. During the prior year, pain became constant and aggravated; pain relief was reported after oral nonsteroidal anti-inflammatory medications. Routine laboratory investigations, including complete blood cell count, erythrocyte

---

[a] First Department of Orthopaedics, Athens University Medical School, 41, Ventouri Street, 15562 Holargos, Athens, Greece
[b] Third Department of Orthopaedics, Athens University Medical School, 2, Nikis, 14561, Kifissia, Athens, Greece
* Corresponding author.
E-mail address: andreasfmavrogenis@yahoo.gr

Clin Podiatr Med Surg 27 (2010) 629–634
doi:10.1016/j.cpm.2010.06.009
0891-8422/10/$ – see front matter © 2010 Elsevier Inc. All rights reserved.

podiatric.theclinics.com

sedimentation rate, C-reactive protein, and complete serum chemistry, were within normal limits.

Lateral radiograph of the right ankle joint showed a small spur and a bony lesion at the talar neck (*Fig. 1*). Bone scan showed increased radioisotope uptake in the left foot, at the head and neck of the talus. (CT scan of the right foot showed a 1.5-cm diameter sclerotic lesion located at the anterior region of the talar neck (*Fig. 2*). MRI showed a low-signal T1-weighted lesion at the right talar neck; the lesion showed high-signal intensity at T2-weighted images. The articular capsule and periarticular soft tissues were thickened and edematous. Bone marrow edema was noticed at the talar neck (*Fig. 3*). Needle biopsy was performed that, however, was not diagnostic.

Through the anterolateral approach, the articular capsule was incised and the lesion was identified on the anterior region of the talar neck. The lesion was loosely attached to bone, and was totally excised without interfering with the adjacent bone. Histologic sections of the excised specimen showed osteoid osteoma (*Fig. 4*).

Patient's recovery was uneventful. Ankle pain resolved immediately postoperatively and did not recur at the latest follow-up examination, 1 year after the operation.

DISCUSSION

First described by Jaffe[7] in 1935, osteoid osteomas are common, benign, osteoblastic bone tumors. The tumors are more common in men than women, and although 75% occur between 5 and 25 years of age, they may occur in the mature skeleton up to 70 years of age. Juxta-articular lesions are characterized by lymphoproliferative synovitis with multiple lymphoid follicles indistinguishable from rheumatoid arthritis. The local periosteal reaction sometimes seen at a distance from a juxta-articular osteoid osteoma is probably, as in rheumatoid arthritis, secondary to the associated synovitis. Panus formation, destruction, and ankylosis of the joint, however, do not occur.[8–23]

Atypical clinical presentation of juxta-articular osteoid osteomas, including nonspecific pain, stiffness, swelling, effusion, synovitis, muscular atrophy, joint contracture, and local warmth, may lead to delayed diagnosis or misdiagnosis.[2–7] Injury has been sometimes correlated with the onset of symptoms and this can make the diagnosis even more difficult, as in the case patient, who was initially

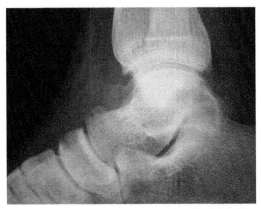

Fig. 1. Lateral radiograph of the right ankle show a small spur and a bony lesion with irregularity of the anterior cortex of the neck of the talus.

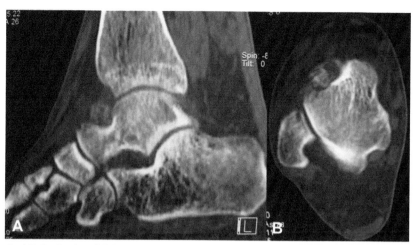

Fig. 2. (*A*) Sagittal and (*B*) axial CT scans of the right ankle joint show a 1.5-cm diameter, well-demarcated bony lesion and surrounding periosteitis at the anterior region of the talar neck.

misdiagnosed with ankle sprain and anterior ankle impingement. Most of the diagnostic problems derive from the atypical radiographic findings. Plain radiographs are often inadequate for the diagnosis of osteoid osteomas of the talus; the nidus of juxta-articular osteoid osteomas is often not shown.[2,4,6] Occasionally, plain radiographs may reveal juxta-articular osteopenia and/or osteoarthritic changes.[24] Technetium-99m bone scan usually does not show intense accumulation of the radioisotope (the nidus) surrounded by an area of low accumulation (the nest); radioisotope activity is often generalized within the joint due to associated synovitis and hyperaemia.[25] In the case patient, foot juxta-articular localization, previous trauma, and low index of suspicion of the physicians who initially investigated and treated the patient misled and delayed the correct diagnosis.

Thin sections of CT scans is the imaging modality of choice for osteoid osteomas, including juxta-articular lesions, showing a low attenuation nidus with internal central

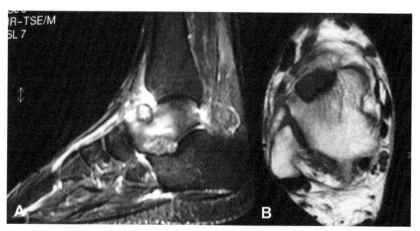

Fig. 3. (*A*) Sagittal T2-weighted MRI shows a high-signal intensity lesion at the anterior talar neck. (*B*) The lesion has a low-signal intensity on T1-weighted MRI.

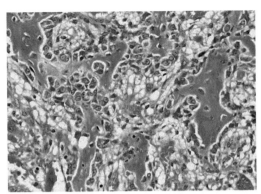

Fig. 4. High-power histologic sections of the excised lesion shows irregular bone trabeculae bordered by osteoblasts (stain, hematoxylin-eosin; original magnification, ×200).

calcification that relates to the maturity and age of the tumor and variable surrounding perinidal sclerosis.[3,4,6] MRI is more expensive and less sensitive than CT scan for accurately identifying a particularly small nidus, but it can be helpful in confirming the diagnosis or ruling out other lesions.[1,6,25]

In the case patient, a clear association between ankle injury and the onset of osteoid osteoma was not established. Because of the absence of an earlier examination, it was impossible to say if the lesion existed or it occurred accidentally after trauma. It may be assumed that ankle sprain may have acted as trigger and activated a silent tumor already present. Ankle sprain and interosseous ligament strain may have caused micro-lesion of the bone around a silent lesion and, with the high vascularity that followed the injury and physiotherapeutic treatment, may have supported an increased production and release of prostaglandins and other pain mediators by the nidus.[18]

Current treatment for osteoid osteomas include minimally invasive techniques, such as percutaneous trephine or drill resection, with or without subsequent injection of ethanol, and thermal destruction with laser photocoagulation or radiofrequency ablation of the nidus.[23,26,27] Surgery is the standard treatment, however, in cases where histology is in doubt, as in the case patient; when neurovascular structures are within 1.5 cm; or with repeated failure of any other minimally invasive ablative technique or percutaneous resection. Clinical success of surgery ranges from 88% to 100%. After excision of the nidus, the synovial inflammation settles and a normal range of joint motion eventually returns.[28]

In conclusion, osteoid osteoma of the talus is an infrequent cause of pain in the ankle, and should be considered in the differential diagnosis of persistent ankle pain in teenagers and young adults who do not respond to treatment directed at more common conditions.

REFERENCES

1. Allen SD, Saifuddin A. Imaging of intra-articular osteoid osteoma. Clin Radiol 2003;58:845–52.
2. Barca F, Leti AA, Spina V. Intra-articular osteoid osteoma of the lower extremity: diagnostic problems. Foot Ankle Int 2002;23(3):264–7.
3. Christodoulou A, Ploumis A, Karkavelas G, et al. A rare case of juxtaarticular osteoid osteoma of the calcaneus initially misdiagnosed as juvenile chronic arthritis. Arthritis Rheum 2003;48(3):776–9.

4. Khurana JS, Mayo-Smith W, Kattapuram SV. Subtalar arthralgia caused by juxtaarticular osteoid osteoma. Clin Orthop Relat Res 1990;252:205–8.
5. Franceschi F, Marinozzi A, Rizzello G, et al. Computed tomography-guided and arthroscopically controlled en bloc retrograde resection of a juxta-articular osteoid osteoma of the tibial plateau. Arthroscopy 2005;21(3):351–9.
6. Georgoulis AD, Papageorgiou CD, Moebius UG, et al. The diagnostic dilemma created by osteoid osteoma that presents as knee pain. Arthroscopy 2002; 18(1):32–7.
7. Jaffe HL. Osteoid osteoma. A benign osteoblastic tumor composed of osteoid and atypical bone. Arch Surg 1935;31:709–28.
8. Martini M, Got G, Chalp Z. 4 new cases of osteoid in talus neck. Rev Chir Orthop Reparatrice Appar Mot 1976;62(6):651–7.
9. Panni AS, Maiotti M, Burke J. Osteoid osteoma of the neck of the talus. Am J Sports Med 1989;17(4):584–8.
10. McGuire MH. Osteoid osteoma of the neck of the talus. Am J Sports Med 1990; 18(2):219.
11. Amendola A, Vellet D, Willits K. Osteoid osteoma of the neck of the talus: percutaneous, computed tomography-guided technique for complete excision. Foot Ankle Int 1994;15(8):429–32.
12. Pikoulas C, Mantzikopoulos G, Thanos L, et al. Unusually located osteoid osteomas. Eur J Radiol 1995;20(2):120–5.
13. Resnick RB, Jarolem KL, Sheskier SC, et al. Arthroscopic removal of an osteoid osteoma of the talus: a case report. Foot Ankle Int 1995;16(4):212–5.
14. Snow SW, Sobel M, DiCarlo EF, et al. Chronic ankle pain caused by osteoid osteoma of the neck of the talus. Foot Ankle Int 1997;18(2):98–101.
15. Chuang SY, Wang SJ, Au MK, et al. Osteoid osteoma in the talar neck: a report of two cases. Foot Ankle Int 1998;19(1):44–7.
16. Tüzüner S, Aydin AT. Arthroscopic removal of an osteoid osteoma at the talar neck. Arthroscopy 1998;14(4):405–9.
17. Bojanić I, Orlić D, Ivković A. Arthroscopic removal of a juxtaarticular osteoid osteoma of the talar neck. J Foot Ankle Surg 2003;42(6):359–62.
18. Pogliacomi F, Vaienti E. Misdiagnosed iuxta-articular osteoid osteoma of the calcaneus following an injury. Acta Biomed 2003;74(3):144–50.
19. Yercan HS, Okcu G, Ozalp T, et al. Arthroscopic removal of the osteoid osteoma on the neck of the talus. Knee Surg Sports Traumatol Arthrosc 2004;12(3):246–9.
20. Gunes T, Erdem M, Sen C, et al. Arthroscopic removal of a subperiosteal osteoid osteoma of the talus. J Am Podiatr Med Assoc 2007;97(3):238–43.
21. Morbidi M, Ventura A, Della Rocca C. Arthroscopic assisted resection of juxtaarticular osteoid osteoma. J Foot Ankle Surg 2007;46(6):470–3.
22. David P, Legname M, Dupond M. Arthroscopic removal of an osteoid osteoma of the talar neck. Orthop Traumatol Surg Res 2009;95(6):454–7.
23. Papagelopoulos PJ, Mavrogenis AF, Kyriakopoulos CK, et al. Radiofrequency ablation of intra-articular osteoid osteoma of the hip. J Int Med Res 2006;34(5):537–44.
24. Norman A, Abdelwabah IF, Buyon J, et al. Osteoid osteoma of the hip stimulating an early onset of osteoarthritis. Radiology 1986;158:417–20.
25. Goldman AB, Schneider R, Pavlov H. Osteoid osteomas of the femoral neck: report of four cases evaluated with isotopic bone scanning, CT and MRI. Radiology 1993;186:227–32.
26. Papagelopoulos PJ, Mavrogenis AF, Galanis EC, et al. Minimally invasive techniques in orthopaedic oncology: radiofrequency and laser thermal ablation. Orthopedics 2005;28(6):563–8.

27. Kyriakopoulos CK, Mavrogenis AF, Pappas J, et al. Percutaneous computed tomography-guided radiofrequency ablation of osteoid osteomas. Eur J Orthop Surg Traumatol 2007;17(1):29–36.
28. Cantwell CP, Obyrne J, Eustace S. Current trends in treatment of osteoid osteoma with an emphasis on radiofrequency ablation. Eur Radiol 2004;14(4):607–17.

Concomitant Acute Osteomyelitis and Squamous Cell Carcinoma of the Foot: A Case Report

Sean Kersh, DPM[a], Shirmeen Lakhani, DPM[a],
Crystal L. Ramanujam, DPM[a], Francis Derk, DPM[b],
Thomas Zgonis, DPM, FACFAS[a],*

KEYWORDS

- Squamous cell carcinoma • Foot • Tumor
- Metastasis • Surgery

Squamous cell carcinoma (SCC) is the second most common type of skin cancer, affecting mostly men and whites, and frequently occurs in sun-exposed areas of the body.[1,2] SCC is a malignancy that can be isolated to local tissues, spread to lymph nodes, or metastasize to distant sites, such as the lungs.[1] In 1835, Hawkins was the first to document the presence of SCC arising in chronic osteomyelitis.[3] SCC has been known to occur in 1.6% to 23% of all patients with chronic osteomyelitis, whereas 85% of these involve the lower extremity, in particular the tibia.[4,5] The typical picture of SCC in the lower extremity includes a painful, draining ulceration of several months' or years' duration with radiographic findings of osseous destruction.[6] Biopsy of these suspicious lesions is essential for appropriate diagnosis and treatment.[7,8] In contrast to several previous reports of SCC in chronic osteomyelitis of the foot, this article presents a rare case of SCC found in the presence of acute osteomyelitis of the toe.

CASE REPORT

A 62-year-old white man presented to the authors' outpatient clinic for evaluation of a red, ulcerated right fifth toe. The patient related prior history of blunt trauma to

[a] Division of Podiatric Medicine and Surgery, Department of Orthopaedic Surgery, The University of Texas Health Science Center at San Antonio, 7703 Floyd Curl Drive – MSC 7776, San Antonio, TX 78229, USA
[b] Podiatry Division, Department of Surgery, Audie L Murphy VA Hospital, San Antonio, TX, USA
* Corresponding author.
E-mail address: zgonis@uthscsa.edu

Clin Podiatr Med Surg 27 (2010) 635–641
doi:10.1016/j.cpm.2010.06.010
0891-8422/10/$ – see front matter © 2010 Elsevier Inc. All rights reserved.

the right foot 1 year before his visit but more recently had treated the toe for what he thought was a wart for approximately 3 weeks. He reported using over-the-counter acid solution to the area but noticed gradual progression to an open wound with redness. Past medical history was significant for chronic obstructive pulmonary disease and 30-pack-year tobacco use.

Physical examination revealed a 1.3 × 1.0 × 0.3 cm superficial granular ulceration to the medial right fifth digit with periwound erythema. Neurovascular status was intact to both feet. Initial plain radiographs showed no evidence of osseous involvement. Due to the superficial nature of the wound, local wound care with the use of a surgical shoe and light duty from work was recommended; however, the patient refused and continued full time as a service technician wearing combat boots. Four weeks later, the wound had worsened, increasing in size with fibrotic tissue, erythema, white chalky drainage, malodor, and probing to bone. Subsequent radiographic evaluation of the right foot demonstrated progressive destruction to the proximal and middle phalanges of fifth digit with severe soft tissue swelling (**Fig. 1**).

Due to the extent of involvement, amputation of the digit was deemed necessary and the patient provided informed consent. All preoperative diagnostic testing was within normal limits. Surgery consisted of sharp disarticulation of the fifth digit from the metatarsophalangeal joint and primary wound closure. Intraoperatively, white chalky material with soft, porous bone and strong malodor were found within the toe. Histopathologic inspection of the tissue showed a well to moderately differentiated invasive SCC extending close to but not into the bone (**Figs. 2–4**). Acute and chronic osteomyelitis of the proximal and middle phalanges with sinus tract was also reported.

The oncology service was consulted for comanagement due to the typically aggressive nature of this neoplasm and concern for metastasis. Full oncologic workup was performed, including CT and positron emission tomography (PET) scans of the abdomen, pelvis, thorax, and chest. The only positive finding was hepatosplenomegaly, which was unrelated to the SCC. There were no signs of lymphadenopathy. Due to the localized nature of the lesion without evidence of metastasis, wide resection of the affected skin was recommended. Mohs surgical technique was then used for adequate resection.[5] This method involves excision of the lesion in question using a dermagraphic map, along with orientation of the lesion in relation to its borders and depth. After each surgical removal of tissue, the specimen is processed, cut on the cryostat and placed on slides, stained, and then read by the Mohs pathologist who examines the sections for malignant cells. If malignancy is found, its location is marked on the map and the surgeon removes the indicated tissue from the patient. This procedure is repeated until no further malignancy is found, thereby ensuring complete removal of the involved tissue. The remaining wound was then closed primarily with nylon suture under minimal tension.

Postoperative care comprised non–weight bearing with a surgical shoe for 3 weeks, followed by suture removal and weight bearing to tolerance with return to full-time work. At 16 months' postoperatively, the patient had no evidence of further infection or recurrence of malignancy.

DISCUSSION

Chronic wounds affected by aggressive SCC have been referred to as Marjolin ulcer, which can result from burn injuries, venous ulcers, and ulcers from osteomyelitis.[9] SCC arising from chronic osteomyelitis has been classically described in the literature for more than 150 years.[10] In the lower extremity, the tibia is the most commonly affected site, followed by the femur and the foot.[4] Ziets and colleagues[11] described successful treatment of a case involving the hallux. Separate reports by Kaplansky

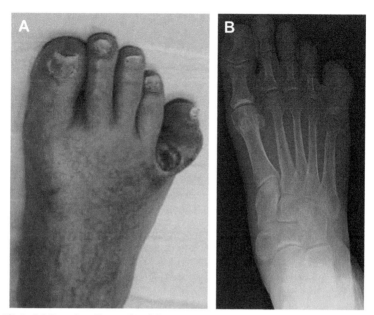

Fig. 1. Clinical (*A*) and radiographic (*B*) pictures of the right foot showing the ulcerated lesion and bony destruction of the right fifth digit.

and colleagues[12] and Patel and colleagues[13] described SCC of the toe masquerading as osteomyelitis, emphasizing the importance of diagnosis with biopsy. In cases of chronic osteomyelitis, the onset of SCC is usually much later than the diagnosis of initial infection, documented as early as 18 months to as late as 64 years.[10] The authors' case report is in stark contrast to these reports and is the first to their knowledge showing SCC in the presence of acute osteomyelitis of the toe.

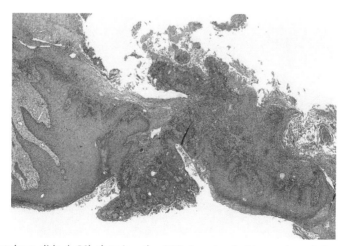

Fig. 2. Histology slide (×20) showing the SCC, invasive (*mid-upper*), well to moderately differentiated. In addition, there is squamous hyperplasia (*left*) with marked acute and chronic inflammation.

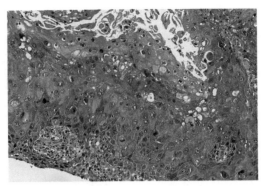

Fig. 3. Histology slide showing the atypical keratinocytes with nuclear pleomorphism, multiple mitosis, and dyskeratosis (original magnification ×200).

The patient was male, in the sixth decade of age, and white, which are all typical characteristics of SCC. The cause of SCC in the presence of osteomyelitis is known to be related to inflammation leading to a local increase in growth factors, which are capable of inducing cellular events of malignant transformation.[6] SCC originates from the squamous epithelium of the surface epidermis and may show varying degrees of differentiation. The clinical appearance of the tumor varies, ranging from a skin-colored, red, or brown nodule with or without scaling to an induration, plaque, exophytic growth, or an ulcerated lesion, as seen with the patient.[14] Gillis and Lee[15] reported that in reference to malignancy, the duration of osteomyelitis is a more critical contributing factor than the age of a patient. The patient did report a remote history of blunt trauma to the toe but that was unrelated to the wound or acute osteomyelitis found on initial presentation to the authors' institution. Differential diagnosis for SCC of the foot due to its clinical appearance may include basal cell carcinoma, Bowen disease, cutaneous granulomas, psoriasis, eczema, and keratoacanthomas.[16]

Diagnosis of acute osteomyelitis in the patient was clear based on clinical findings and associated radiographic evidence of osseous destruction to the toe.

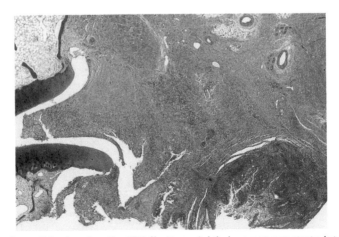

Fig. 4. Histology slide showing the SCC (*bottom right*) does not penetrate into the bone (*upper left*). There is marked acute and chronic inflammation in the soft tissue extending into the articular space (original magnification ×20).

Radiographically, SCC may also demonstrate replacement of bone with the presence of an invasive soft tissue mass.[13] MRI is also useful for diagnosis of SCC to differentiate it from other soft tissue neoplasms.[14] Definitive diagnosis is made through shave biopsy, punch biopsy, incisional biopsy, or excisional biopsy of the lesion. Histologically, SCC is characterized by an intraepidermal proliferation of atypical keratinocytes.[1] Once diagnosis is confirmed, suspicion for metastasis can be ruled out using full-body PET and CT scans, because the most common site for distant metastasis is the lungs.[10] Generally, amputation proximal to the lesion is the treatment of choice for both acute osteomyelitis and SCC. In the case report, amputation of the fifth

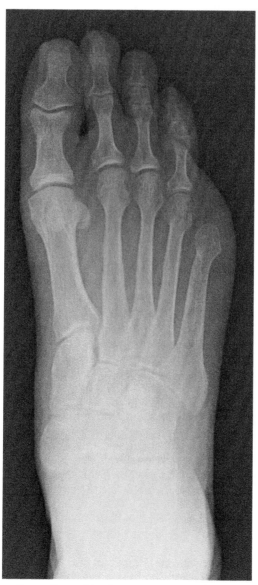

Fig. 5. Final postoperative radiographic picture at 1.5 years' follow-up.

toe was modified through the use of Mohs micrographic surgical technique. Goldberg and Arbesfeld[17] first described this method for excision of SCC arising in chronic osteomyelitis. Kirsner and colleagues[5] also reported on this technique as a limb-sparing option for cases involving the tibia. Advantages of this surgical technique compared with other options for treating cutaneous neoplasms include superior cure rates and maximal tissue conservation.[18] Long-term surveillance for recurrence or metastasis is imperative to patient survival. At 1.5 years' follow-up both by the authors' service and the oncology service, the patient showed no evidence of recurrent SCC or infection (**Fig. 5**).

The case emphasizes that surgeons should include SCC in their differential diagnosis for recalcitrant ulcerations in the setting of acute osteomyelitis of the foot. Although concurrence of these disease processes is rare and may complicate matters, the case illustrates that a successful functional outcome is possible with high index of suspicion, accurate diagnosis, and effective surgical management.

ACKNOWLEDGMENTS

The authors would like to thank Alma J. Sanchez-Salazar, MD, for her help with the histopathological analysis.

REFERENCES

1. Johnson TM, Rowe DE, Nelson BR, et al. Squamous cell carcinoma of the skin (excluding lip and oral mucosa). J Am Acad Dermatol 1992;26:467–84.
2. Leiter U, Garbe C. Epidemiology of melanoma and nonmelanoma skin cancer—the role of sunlight. Adv Exp Med Biol 2008;624:89–103.
3. Hawkins C. Cases of warty tumours in cicatrices. Med Chir Trans 1835;19:19.
4. Altay M, Arikan M, Yildiz Y, et al. Squamous cell carcinoma arising in chronic osteomyelitis in foot and ankle. Foot Ankle Int 2004;25:805–9.
5. Kirsner RS, Spencer J, Falanga V, et al. Squamous cell carcinoma arising in osteomyelitis and chronic wounds. Treatment with Mohs micrographic surgery vs amputation. Dermatol Surg 1996;22:1015–8.
6. Wangner RF, Grande DJ. Pseudoepitheliomatous hyperplasia vs. squamous cell carcinoma arising from chronic osteomyelitis of the humerus. J Dermatol Surg Oncol 1986;12:632–5.
7. McGrory JE, Pritchard DJ, Unni KK, et al. Malignant lesions arising in chronic osteomyelitis. Clin Orthop 1999;362:181–9.
8. Johnson LL, Kempson RL. Epidermoid carcinoma in chronic osteomyelitis: diagnostic problems and management: report of ten cases. J Bone Joint Surg Am 1965;47:133–45.
9. Smidt LS, Smidt LF, Chedid MB, et al. Radical surgical treatment for Marjolin ulcer occurring after chronic osteomyelitis. South Med J 2005;98:1053.
10. Laffosse JM, Bensafi H, Accadbled F, et al. Squamous-cell carcinoma and osteomyelitis: three cases and a review of the literature. Rev Chir Orthop Reparatrice Appar Mot 2007;93:72–7.
11. Ziets RJ, Evanski PM, Lusskin R, et al. Squamous cell carcinoma complicating chronic osteomyelitis in a toe: a case report and review of the literature. Foot Ankle 1991;12:178–81.
12. Kaplansky DB, Kademian ME, VanCourt RB. Metastatic squamous cell carcinoma resembling cellulitis and osteomyelitis of the fifth toe. J Foot Ankle Surg 2006;45:182–4.

13. Patel A, Ryan JF, Badrinath K, et al. Squamous cell carcinoma of the toe masquerading as osteomyelitis. J R Soc Med 1988;81:418–20.
14. Theodorou SJ, Theodorou DJ, Bona SJ, et al. Primary squamous cell carcinoma: an incidental toe mass. Am J Roentgenol 2005;184:S110–1.
15. Gillis L, Lee S. Cancer as a sequel to war wounds. J Bone Joint Surg Br 1951;33: 167–79.
16. Potter BK, Pitcher JD Jr, Adams SC, et al. Squamous cell carcinoma of the foot. Foot Ankle Int 2009;30:517–23.
17. Goldberg DJ, Arbesfeld D. Squamous cell carcinoma arising in a site of chronic osteomyelitis. Treatment with Mohs micrographic surgery. J Dermatol Surg Oncol 1991;17:788–90.
18. Ramanujam CL, Lakhani S, Derk F, et al. Cutaneous non-Hodgkin's lymphoma of the foot: a rare case report. J Foot Ankle Surg 2009;48:581–4.

Index

Note: Page numbers of article titles are in **boldface** type.

Clin Podiatr Med Surg 27 (2010) 643–654
doi:10.1016/S0891-8422(10)00075-3
0891-8422/10/$ – see front matter © 2010 Elsevier Inc. All rights reserved.

podiatric.theclinics.com

United States Postal Service

Statement of Ownership, Management, and Circulation
(All Periodicals Publications Except Requestor Publications)

1. Publication Title
Clinics in Podiatric Medicine & Surgery

2. Publication Number
0 0 0 – 7 0 7

3. Filing Date
9/15/10

4. Issue Frequency
Jan, Apr, Jul, Oct

5. Number of Issues Published Annually
4

6. Annual Subscription Price
$252.00

7. Complete Mailing Address of Known Office of Publication (Not printer) (Street, city, county, state, and ZIP+4®)

Elsevier Inc.
360 Park Avenue South
New York, NY 10010-1710

Contact Person
Stephen Bushing

Telephone (Include area code)
215-239-3688

8. Complete Mailing Address of Headquarters or General Business Office of Publisher (Not printer)

Elsevier Inc., 360 Park Avenue South, New York, NY 10010-1710

9. Full Names and Complete Mailing Addresses of Publisher, Editor, and Managing Editor (Do not leave blank)

Publisher (Name and complete mailing address)

Kim Murphy, Elsevier, Inc., 1600 John F. Kennedy Blvd. Suite 1800, Philadelphia, PA 19103-2899

Editor (Name and complete mailing address)

Patrick Manley, Elsevier, Inc., 1600 John F. Kennedy Blvd. Suite 1800, Philadelphia, PA 19103-2899

Managing Editor (Name and complete mailing address)

Catherine Bewick, Elsevier, Inc., 1600 John F. Kennedy Blvd. Suite 1800, Philadelphia, PA 19103-2899

10. Owner (Do not leave blank. If the publication is owned by a corporation, give the name and address of the corporation immediately followed by the names and addresses of all stockholders owning or holding 1 percent or more of the total amount of stock. If not owned by a corporation, give the names and addresses of the individual owners. If owned by a partnership or other unincorporated firm, give its name and address as well as those of each individual owner. If the publication is published by a nonprofit organization, give its name and address.)

Full Name	Complete Mailing Address
Wholly owned subsidiary of	4520 East-West Highway
Reed/Elsevier, US holdings	Bethesda, MD 20814

11. Known Bondholders, Mortgagees, and Other Security Holders Owning or Holding 1 Percent or More of Total Amount of Bonds, Mortgages, or Other Securities. If none, check box ☐ None

Full Name	Complete Mailing Address
N/A	

12. Tax Status (For completion by nonprofit organizations authorized to mail at nonprofit rates) (Check one)
The purpose, function, and nonprofit status of this organization and the exempt status for federal income tax purposes:
☐ Has Not Changed During Preceding 12 Months
☐ Has Changed During Preceding 12 Months (Publisher must submit explanation of change with this statement)

PS Form 3526, September 2007 (Page 1 of 3 (instructions Page 3)) PSN 7530-01-000-9931 PRIVACY NOTICE: See our Privacy policy in www.usps.com

---

13. Publication Title
Clinics in Podiatric Medicine & Surgery

14. Issue Date for Circulation Data Below
April 2010

15. Extent and Nature of Circulation

		Average No. Copies Each Issue During Preceding 12 Months	No. Copies of Single Issue Published Nearest to Filing Date
a. Total Number of Copies (Net press run)		1321	1250
b. Paid Circulation (By Mail and Outside the Mail)	(1) Mailed Outside-County Paid Subscriptions Stated on PS Form 3541. (Include paid distribution above nominal rate, advertiser's proof copies, and exchange copies)	776	724
	(2) Mailed In-County Paid Subscriptions Stated on PS Form 3541 (Include paid distribution above nominal rate, advertiser's proof copies, and exchange copies)		
	(3) Paid Distribution Outside the Mails Including Sales Through Dealers and Carriers, Street Vendors, Counter Sales, and Other Paid Distribution Outside USPS®	62	61
	(4) Paid Distribution by Other Classes Mailed Through the USPS (e.g. First-Class Mail®)		
c. Total Paid Distribution (Sum of 15b (1), (2), (3), and (4))		838	785
d. Free or Nominal Rate Distribution (By Mail and Outside the Mail)	(1) Free or Nominal Rate Outside-County Copies Included on PS Form 3541	81	78
	(2) Free or Nominal Rate In-County Copies Included on PS Form 3541		
	(3) Free or Nominal Rate Copies Mailed at Other Classes Through the USPS (e.g. First-Class Mail)		
	(4) Free or Nominal Rate Distribution Outside the Mail (Carriers or other means)		
e. Total Free or Nominal Rate Distribution (Sum of 15d (1), (2), (3) and (4))		81	78
f. Total Distribution (Sum of 15c and 15e)		919	863
g. Copies not Distributed (See instructions to publishers #4 (page #3))		402	387
h. Total (Sum of 15f and g)		1321	1250
i. Percent Paid (15c divided by 15f times 100)		91.19%	90.96%

16. Publication of Statement of Ownership
☐ If the publication is a general publication, publication of this statement is required. Will be printed in the **October 2010** issue of this publication.
☐ Publication not required

17. Signature and Title of Editor, Publisher, Business Manager, or Owner

Stephen R. Bushing — Fulfillment/Inventory Specialist

Date
September 15, 2010

I certify that all information furnished on this form is true and complete. I understand that anyone who furnishes false or misleading information on this form or who omits material or information requested on the form may be subject to criminal sanctions (including fines and imprisonment) and/or civil sanctions (including civil penalties).

PS Form 3526, September 2007 (Page 2 of 3)

Moving?

Make sure your subscription moves with you!

To notify us of your new address, find your **Clinics Account Number** (located on your mailing label above your name), and contact customer service at:

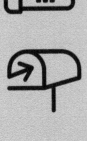

Email: journalscustomerservice-usa@elsevier.com

800-654-2452 (subscribers in the U.S. & Canada)
314-447-8871 (subscribers outside of the U.S. & Canada)

Fax number: 314-447-8029

Elsevier Health Sciences Division
Subscription Customer Service
3251 Riverport Lane
Maryland Heights, MO 63043

*To ensure uninterrupted delivery of your subscription, please notify us at least 4 weeks in advance of move.